# Public Health Nursing

## Scope and Standards of Practice,

### 3rd Edition

D0879698

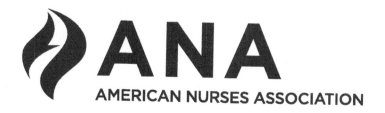

AMERICAN NURSES ASSOCIATION

The American Nurses Association (ANA) is a national professional association. This publication reflects the position of ANA regarding the scope and standards of public health nursing practice and should be reviewed in conjunction with state board of nursing regulations. State law, rules, and regulations govern the practice of nursing, *while Public Health Nursing: Scope and Standards of Practice, 3rd Edition* guides registered nurses in the application of their professional skills and responsibilities.

## About the American Nurses Association

The American Nurses Association (ANA) is the only full-service professional organization representing the interests of the nation's 4.2 million registered nurses through its constituent/state nurses associations and its organizational affiliates. The ANA advances the nursing profession by fostering high standards of nursing practice, promoting the rights of nurses in the workplace, projecting a positive and realistic view of nursing, and by lobbying the Congress and regulatory agencies on health care issues affecting nurses and the public.

American Nurses Association
8515 Georgia Avenue, Suite 400
Silver Spring, MD 20910

Library of Congress Cataloging-in-Publication Data

Names: American Nurses Association, issuing body.
Title: Public health nursing : scope and standards of practice / American Nurses Association.
Other titles: Public health nursing (American Nurses Association)
Description: Third edition. | Silver Spring, MD : American Nurses Association, [2022] | Includes bibliographical references and index.
Identifiers: LCCN 2022013995 (print) | LCCN 2022013996 (ebook) | ISBN 9781953985002 (paperback) | ISBN 9781953985019 (adobe pdf) | ISBN 9781953985026 (epub) | ISBN 9781953985033 (mobi)
Subjects: MESH: Public Health Nursing--standards | Community Health Nursing | Nurse's Role | United States | Guideline
Classification: LCC RT97 (print) | LCC RT97 (ebook) | NLM WY 108 | DDC 610.73/4--dc23/eng/20220412
LC record available at https://lccn.loc.gov/2022013995
LC ebook record available at https://lccn.loc.gov/2022013996    610.73/4--dc23/ eng/20220412
LC record available at https://lccn.loc.gov/2022013995
LC ebook record available at https://lccn.loc.gov/2022013996

SAN: 851-3481

# Contents

# Contributors

*Public Health Nursing: Scope and Standards of Practice, Third Edition*, is the product of extensive thought work by a volunteer group of public health registered nurses from both practice and academic environments. Workgroup members began their review and revision efforts in November 2018 by examining the American Nurses Association's (ANA) *Public Health Nursing: Scope and Standards of Practice, Second Edition* (2013); *Nursing: Scope and Standards of Practice, Third Edition* (ANA, 2015b); Quad Council Coalition Competency Review Task Force's *Community/Public Health Nursing Competencies* (2018); and extensive public health nursing, public health, and other publications and resources. This new scope and standards document originated from the multitude of decisions garnered during a significant number of video telephone conference calls and email communications of the diverse workgroup members in 2018–2021.

The document was finalized after three review steps. The first review involved a 30-day public comment period in April–May 2021, followed by all workgroup members examining every submitted comment, resulting in further workgroup refinements of the draft document. The two following official ANA review processes included evaluation by the Committee on Nursing Practice Standards in November 2021 and final review and approval by the ANA Board of Directors in December 2021.

## Public Health Nursing Scope and Standards Revision Workgroup Members

Susan Little, DNP, RN, PHNA-BC, CPH, CPM, FAAN, Co-chairperson

Susan "Sue" M. Swider, PhD, RN, PHNA-BC, FAAN, Co-chairperson

Kathleen M. Andresen, DNP, RN, CNE

Diane Arcilla, DNP, RN

Rosemary V. Chaudry, PhD, MPH, MHA, APHN-BC, PHCNS-BC, CPH, CNL

Jennifer L. Cooper, DNP, RN, PHNA-BC, CNE

Kim A. Decker, PhD, RN, CNS

Lori Edwards, DrPH, MPH, BSN, RN, CNS-PCH, BC

Juanita C. Graham, DNP, RN, FRSPH

Alisa R. Haushalter, DNP, RN, PHNA-BC

Joni L. Hensley, BSN, RN-BC, CIC

Kirk Koyama, MSN, RN, PHN, CNS

Jennifer L. Morton, DNP, MPH, PHNA-BC

Karen N. Ouzts, PhD, RN, PHNA-BC

Angeleta "Zippy" Robinson, DNP, CNL, LSSGB

Christine W. Saltzberg, PhD, MSHCE, MS, PHCNS-BC, RN

Claudia M. Smith, PhD, MPH, RN

Florence M. Weierbach, PhD, MPH, MSN, RN

## ANA Committee on Nursing Practice Standards

Elizabeth "Liz" O. Dietz, EdD, RN, CS-NP, CSN (Co-Chair)

Mona Pearl Treyball, PhD, RN, CNS, CCRN-K, FAAN (Co-Chair)

Nena M. Bonuel, PhD, RN, APRN-BC, ACNS-BC, CCRN-K

Patricia Bowe, DNP, MS, RN

Danette Culver, MSN, RN, APRN, ACNS-BC, CCRN-K

Tonette "Toni" McAndrew, MPA, RN

Linda Inez Perkins, MSN, RN-BC

Michael Manasia, MSN, RN, OCN (Alternate)

Shelly Wells, PhD, MBA, APRN-CNS, ANEF (Alternate)

## ANA Staff

Carol J. Bickford, PhD, RN-BC, CPHIMS, FAMIA, FHIMSS, FAAN, Content Editor

Katie Boston-Leary, PhD, MBA, MHA, RN, NEA-BC, Contributor

Erin Walpole, BA, PMP, Production Editor

James Angelo, MA, Director of Publications

# Public Health Nursing Scope of Practice

## INTRODUCTION

Public health nursing (PH nursing) addresses the health of all people/ populations within communities for the purpose of social betterment. Social betterment, a term first used by Lillian Wald in 1912 to describe PH nursing, is attained by considering the upstream or precursor determinants of health in the places where people live, work, learn, play, and worship. Public health nurses (PHNs) seek to ensure health equity and well-being for populations by working to prevent and reduce health disparities. PH nursing practice is population-based, and care can be focused on and across multiple levels—individuals, families/small groups, communities, and systems—but always within the context of the community as a whole (Minnesota Department of Health, 2019).

For more than a century, PH nursing has significantly contributed to the population's health by bringing together nursing knowledge and skills with public health expertise (Kneipp et al, 2011; Kneipp et al., 2013; Monsen et al., 2010; Monsen et al., 2011; Monsen et al, 2017; Olsen et al., 2018; Swider et al., 2017). PHNs work to create effective partnerships to address health and its determinants. Beginning in the early 20th century, Lillian Wald and Lavinia Dock partnered with their nursing colleagues at the Henry Street Settlement House in New York City's Lower East Side. Their spirited innovation and organization supported their collaboration with communities to heal, mobilize, support, and bring about change among the disadvantaged populations with whom they lived and worked. Such partnerships continue today as PHNs work with communities, organizations, and populations to identify public health assets and address public health needs at both the level of the community and of the health care and policy formation systems.

Nurses educated and practicing in public health are well positioned to lead all nurses to make the changes being sought for population health in the 21st century (Gorski et al., 2019; Pittman, 2019; Public Health Foundation [PHF], 2019; Storfjell et al., 2017). PHNs have the knowledge, skills, and abilities to lead the nursing profession in creating healthier communities, as called for during the creation of *The Future of Nursing 2030* (National Academies of Sciences, Engineering, and Medicine [NASEM], 2021). As leaders in public and population health, PHNs promote a culture of health by improving the health of individuals, families, and communities and by reducing health inequities through public health interventions, advocacy, and policy development (*The Future of Nursing 2020–2030*, 2021).

# DEFINITION OF PUBLIC HEALTH NURSING

The current definition of PH nursing is adapted from the 2013 Public Health Nursing Section of the American Public Health Association resource, "The Definition and Practice of Public Health Nursing":

- Public health nursing is the practice of promoting and protecting the health of populations using knowledge from nursing, social, and public health sciences. (American Public Health Association [APHA], Public Health Nursing Section, 2013)
- The PH nursing specialty employs all levels of prevention, with an emphasis on primary prevention. PH nursing focuses on improving health outcomes by addressing social, physical, environmental, and other determinants of health. PH nursing includes, but is not limited to, assessment, program planning, evaluation, advocacy, outreach, cross-sector collaboration, research, policy development, and assurance. At the levels of individual, family, group, community, population, and systems, PH nursing addresses health through the application of theory and evidence and the creation of multi-sectoral partnerships. PHNs have a commitment to social and environmental justice, health equity, and community well-being.

## Evolution of the Definition of Public Health Nursing

PH nursing has evolved from the days of Lillian Wald to present-day practice. Over time, terms describing PH nursing practice have alternated between PH nursing and community health nursing to accurately describe the focus on health across levels of care, but always within the context of the community. The first known use of the term *public health nursing* is in Lillian Wald's 1912 description of PH nursing as the name for nurses "doing work for social betterment" in any setting (Brainard, 1995; Fitzpatrick, 1975). The term *public* related to "all the people as a whole." By the 1920s, the majority of PHNs were employed by local and state health departments, and the term *public* became associated with "employment by the government."

In the 1960s, the term *community health nurse* emerged to describe nurses working with individuals in community settings, such as home health care or case management. By the turn of the 21st century, however, PHNs identified that community health nursing was related to the setting and did not differentiate the focus of practice. Use of the term *public health nursing* was reinvigorated to describe nursing practice focused on populations, bringing together nursing, public health, and social sciences to guide practice, always within the context of the community, whether at the individual, family/group, community, or system level. The definition above reflects this understanding. (See Appendix A for a history of the definition of PH nursing.)

# CORE CONCEPTS GUIDING PUBLIC HEALTH NURSING PRACTICE

Nursing practice is guided by an array of key concepts, such as caring, nursing process, and ethics. Additional concepts of critical importance in practice, education, and research for the specialty of PH nursing are listed below.

## 1. Social Determinants of Health

The World Health Organization (WHO) defines the Determinants of Health as the conditions in which people are born, grow, live, work, and age (Mahony & Jones, 2013). "Health is influenced by many factors, which may generally be organized into five broad categories known as determinants of health: genetics, behavior, environmental and physical influences, medical care and social factors. These five categories are interconnected. The fifth category, also called social determinants of health (SDOH), encompasses economic and social conditions that influence the health of people and communities" (Centers for Disease Control and Prevention [CDC], 2019, December, 19).

The importance of SDOH in health outcomes has been reinforced by the work of Thomas Frieden in the Health Impact Framework (see Figure 1). Described as a "framework for public health action," the health impact pyramid has five tiers (Frieden, 2010). Two key elements of this framework to improve health are often overlooked: it extends beyond the provision of health care services, and it acknowledges and includes the multiple determinants of health.

What does the Health Impact Framework mean for PH nursing? Starting from the base and moving to the top, the pyramid tiers include actions that are taken to create changes in or affect socioeconomic factors, the environmental context of healthy decisions, long-lasting protection, ongoing care and clinical interventions, and counseling and education. PHNs act to address each level of the pyramid. Frieden contends that "interventions that address [the] social determinants of health have the greatest potential" to benefit the public's health (2010, p. 594). In other words, actions at the bottom of the pyramid are effective at the community/population level and move to more of a focus on individuals as one moves up the tiers.

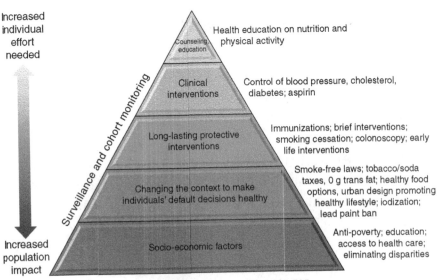

Frieden T. *American Journal of Public Health. 2010;100(4):590-595.*

**Figure 1. Health Impact Pyramid**

PHNs focus on key factors that affect an individual's or community's overall health and ability to respond to disease. These factors include the physical environment, structural racism, poverty, economic inequality, social status, stress, education level, social inequities, employment, social support, and the ability to obtain food and accessible health care (Egede & Walker, 2020; Mahony & Jones, 2013).

PHNs' focus on SDOH helps address larger goals of social and environmental justice and health equity. PHNs recognize the critical role that the environment plays by striving to create physical and social environments that foster positive health outcomes and help expand health-related choices available to individuals within a community. *Healthy People 2020* identifies the value of empowering people toward the goal of achieving positive health outcomes by increasing health promotion and disease prevention activities, such as smoking cessation and healthier diets for people at home, work, and school. (Heffernan et al., 2019). The recently released *Healthy People 2030* continues to increase focus on improving the physical and social environments so necessary for positive health outcomes.

PHNs work to address SDOH by assessing underlying conditions that contribute to inequities in population health outcomes. These determinants shape social hierarchy, resulting in power differences, marginalization, classism, racism, and oppression of selected groups. Research into SDOH, including income, education, race, and gender, often indicates that these are causal factors for health disparities and inequities (Alderwick & Gottlieb, 2019).

Macroeconomic factors, such as public expenditures, taxes, and private savings, are related to policymaking and result in downstream health inequities. Thus, PHNs advocate for changes in the structural societal and political macrolevels. The SDOH framework also outlines and analyzes the intermediate determinants that ultimately influence the material, psychosocial, biological, and behavioral factors of health (World Health Organization [WHO], 2019a).

PHNs also address social needs at the individual level of SDOH, defined as the material resources necessary for physical and mental health and well-being. When addressing social needs, PHNs focus on enhancing circumstances that may facilitate health at the microlevel and support the acquisition of resources such as food, water, and health care. PHNs may also provide social needs support by improving conditions such as inadequate housing.

## 2. Community Collaboration

Based on core competencies of public health practice (PHF, 2014), leadership in the field of public health involves incorporating key principles of collaboration into all interactions with individuals, populations, communities, and organizations (Public Health Leadership Society [PHLS], 2002). Therefore, collaborating with the community at the outset is a precondition for ethical and effective practice, which means that community members (as stakeholders) should be involved in identifying problems and needs, developing programs and policies, and "reconciling" what constitutes the most important concern of the community (Rentmeester & Dasgupta, 2012, p. 236).

This collaboration goes beyond determining the best course of action to include community participation in development, implementation, and evaluation of any interventions. Unless the collaboration process allows for full involvement of representative stakeholders in every decision-making step, the framework of a "fair decision process" conflicts with the ethical principles of public health and PH nursing practice (Marckmann et al., 2015, p. 5). Collaborating with a population or community, according to the standards of both nursing practice and public health (ANA, 2015b; PHLS, 2002), means that community members (stakeholders) should be involved in decision-making processes from beginning to end, including involvement in managing conflicts of interest and competing claims of decision makers and developing and evaluating programs and policies.

## 3. Population Health

The terms *public*, *people*, and *population* have traditionally been used interchangeably in the public health world to address the health of all people. *Population* is defined as "a collection of individuals in a geographically defined area (e.g., town, city, state, region, nation, multinational region), or a group of individuals within the community (such as school students, workers in industry, or persons of similar age)" (ANA, 1986, p. 18). A *community* is a set of people in interaction who may or may not share a sense of place or belonging and who act intentionally for a common purpose (e.g., live in a neighborhood, work at a given company, or share a common cultural or demographic characteristic, health condition, or threat to health) (Ervin & Kulbok, 2018). Examples of communities include immigrant groups, refugees, individuals who have experienced gender discrimination, persons with mental illness, and victims of a disaster.

*Subpopulations* include groups or aggregates within the larger population. Group members usually have face-to-face contact. Aggregates are usually identified by health professionals according to one or more common characteristics; aggregates can consist of people experiencing a specific health condition (e.g., diseases, disabilities, pregnancy), engaging in behaviors that have the potential to negatively affect health (e.g., smoking tobacco, vaping), sharing a common risk factor or risk exposure (asbestos, lead, pesticides exposure), or experiencing an emerging health threat or risk (APHA, 1996).

Recently, the concept of population health has become commonly used across the health care system. *Population health* is defined as "the health outcomes of a group of people, including the distribution of such outcomes within the group" (Kindig & Stoddart, 2003, p. 380). In this conception, populations are aggregates of people with common characteristics that become a focus for care across the continuum. Improving population health, improving the experience of care, and reducing per-capita health care costs are the triple aims of the 2019 Institute for Healthcare Improvement (IHI) framework to improve the US health care system (Institute for Healthcare Improvement [IHI], 2019). Bodenheimer and Sinsky (2014) expand this framework to the Quadruple Aim with the inclusion of improving the work life of health care providers, including clinicians and staff.

Population health includes application of basic public health knowledge and skills across the care continuum. On this continuum, *population health management* or *population management* refers to the management of health outcomes of a clinical population enrolled in a discrete health care system that is held financially accountable (Berwick et al., 2008; Storfjell et al., 2017). At the other end of the population health continuum, broader collaboration of health-related and civic organizations working together improves "…health outcomes for a specific population, with shared accountability and a commitment to addressing upstream determinants of health" (Storfjell et al., 2017, p. 6). Bresnick (2017) clarifies: "Population health is a term more commonly used in the clinical sphere and the health IT industry, while the phrase public health tends to be favored by government officials and the stakeholders who work closely with them."

The recognition that health has multiple determinants, including social, has led to a "resurgence of the population health model that had long been suppressed by the popular medical model" (Radzyminski, 2007, p. 38). With the advent of computers and large data sets of health-related information, knowledge about multiple determinants of health and their interactions has expanded. The shift in studying human health from the broad perspective of multiple determinants of health is a "return to our historical roots" for public health professionals, including PHNs (Kindig & Stoddart, 2003, p. 382).

In 2010, the federal Patient Protection and Affordable Care Act (ACA) required that nonprofit hospitals conduct community health needs assessments (CHNA) and develop implementation strategies to address those needs (ACA, 2010). In response to this mandate, the Public Health Foundation (PHF) published the *Competencies for Population Health Professionals* in March 2019 to strengthen the connection between public health and health care. These competencies are basic skills for health professionals across the care continuum, including those working in hospitals, health systems, public health, and other places engaged in the assessment of population health needs and the development, delivery, and improvement of population health programs, services, and practices, whether for broad populations or targeted populations.

PHNs take basic population health skills to the next level with a focus on the broader context in which people live and how that context enables or hinders health. PHNs have a long history of assessing the needs of individuals, families, and communities; building partnerships across sectors to find solutions; and developing and advocating for upstream solutions (Pittman, 2019). As experts in population health, PHNs offer expertise and support to other nurses and health care providers engaged in offering population health management services.

In 2019, the Minnesota Department of Health clarified that interventions by PHNs are *population-based* if they:

- Focus on entire populations possessing similar health concerns or characteristics;
- Are guided by an assessment of population health status determined through a community health assessment (CHA) process;
- Consider the broad determinants of health;
- Consider all levels of prevention, with a preference for primary prevention; and
- Consider all levels of practice: individual-focused, family-/ group-focused, community-focused, and systems-focused (Minnesota Department of Health, 2019, pp. 13–15).

PHNs are *population-based* and *focus on individual/family, community, and systems* levels when they develop and implement their plans of care.

In a time when "every nurse is a population health nurse," and population health is being integrated throughout nursing curriculums, distinguishable characteristics clearly differentiate the PH nursing specialty from other nursing specialties. PHNs are distinguished by their ability to use analytic community assessment skills to pursue health promotion and prevention, working with communities and populations as equal partners (Kulbok et al., 2012). PHNs collaborate to build partnerships within and outside the health sector and influence mid- and upstream sustainable health interventions focused on primary prevention and health promotion. Additionally, with their emphasis on systems thinking, PHNs can lead health care system changes to ensure that needs are met equitably in all communities (Bekemeier et al., 2014).

# 4. Ecological Model of Health: Micro- to Macro-levels

PHNs, working with individuals, groups, communities, and populations, practice across a continuum of micro-, meso-, and macro levels of society, but always within the population context. At the micro-level, PHNs work with individuals, small groups, and families to address health issues; provide primary, secondary, or tertiary prevention; and emphasize disease prevention and health promotion. At the meso-level, PHNs work with communities or specific populations or groups in society, such as schools, workplaces, or people with common health risks, viewing this level as the focus of care and determining the impact of population-level interactions. PHNs working at the macro-level evaluate and address broader population- or societal-level factors that affect health, such as policies, laws, or interactions between nations (Blackstone, 2012).

The Minnesota Intervention Wheel differentiates interventions by category and level of practice (individual/family, community, or systems), describing the scope of practice by what is similar across settings (Minnesota Department of Health, 2019). These three levels approximate the micro-, meso-, and macro-levels described above. Apart from delegated functions, the interventions described in the Minnesota Intervention Wheel are not exclusive to PH nursing, as they are also used by other public health disciplines, but the breadth of scope and combination of levels are unique to PH nursing practice. The interventions across levels of practice include:

- Surveillance;
- Disease and health event investigation;
- Outreach;
- Screening;
- Case finding;
- Referral and follow-up;
- Case management;
- Delegated functions;
- Health teaching;
- Counseling;

- Consultation;
- Collaboration;
- Coalition building;
- Community organizing;
- Advocacy;
- Social marketing; and
- Policy development and enforcement.

## 5. Culturally Congruent Practice: Respectful, Equitable, and Inclusionary

Culturally congruent practice is the application of evidence-based nursing within the context of the preferred cultural values, beliefs, worldview, and practices of the healthcare consumer, community, and other stakeholders. Society is increasingly multicultural, as characterized by differences in ethnicity, race, social class, education, sexual orientation and gender identity, language, age, religion, and family structures (Murcia & Lopez, 2016). A culturally diverse society requires culturally competent healthcare providers and delivery of care to ensure an acceptance and openness to understanding varying beliefs, traditions, and ethnic practices (Murcia & Lopez, 2016).

Cultural competence represents the process by which PHNs demonstrate culturally congruent practice. To support cultural competence, several elements are needed, including awareness of cultural values, beliefs, and attitudes; openness to understanding and accepting the diversity of people; and skills to combine the awareness and the knowledge to provide culturally appropriate services and effective intercultural communication in cultural encounters (Campinha-Bacote, 2002; Danso, 2018).

*Cultural sensitivity*, an added dimension to providing culturally congruent care, is defined as the ability to be open and responsive to attitudes, feelings, or life circumstances of groups of people who share common distinctive aspects of racial, national, religious, linguistic, or cultural heritage (Office of Minority Health, 2001). PHNs include cultural sensitivity in the practice of caring for diverse populations at all levels, micro to macro (e.g., individual to systems).

Cultural humility extends beyond cultural competence and is another dimension of culturally congruent practice that PHNs must address. "Cultural humility is a humble and respectful attitude toward individuals of other cultures that pushes one to challenge their own cultural biases, realize they cannot possibly know everything about other cultures, and approach learning about other cultures as a life-long goal and process" (Gonzales & Levitas, 2020, as cited in ANA, 2021, p. 23). Engagement in relationships with diverse communities requires a sense of humility, further requiring self-awareness, self-reflection, and self-critique. Cultural humility acknowledges the subjectivity of culture and the lifelong process of learning to engage in meaningful and effective relationships across diverse cultural values, beliefs, and practices (Fisher-Borne et al., 2015).

Cultural safety is a broader concept that has emerged over time. Debate exists as to whether cultural safety represents a continued evolution of the concept of cultural competence or a radically new paradigm. What is clear is that cultural safety goes beyond attaining the knowledge, skills, and attitudes necessary to deliver services to diverse populations. Cultural safety addresses social inequities steeped in power inequities. Cultural safety demands that PHNs and public health organizations that PHNs represent focus on power inequities, including the inherent power inequities between PHNs and individuals, families, and communities served as well as power inequities within the public health system. Achieving equity at the population level necessitates that PHNs practice cultural safety. Cultural safety also demands self-reflection at the individual PHN and organizational levels (Curtis et al., 2019). Culturally congruent PHN practice requires aspects of cultural competence, sensitivity, safety, and humility (Marion et al., 2017).

# 6. Levels of Prevention

The PH nursing specialty employs all levels of prevention (primary, secondary, and tertiary), with an emphasis on primary prevention. This follows assessments at the individual, family, community, and population levels and the development of an understanding of the world in which people live. The primary prevention approach in health care aims to prevent disease or injury before it ever occurs and may include:

- Promoting community education regarding the avoidance of medical and behavioral health risks, such as the mismanagement of prescription drugs, tobacco/e-cigarette use, and poor eating habits;
- Implementing health promotion methods, such as routine immunizations of children, adults, and the elderly; and
- Developing community health programs, such as oral and dental hygiene instruction, for improving the population health (CDC, n.d.-b).

PHNs also serve as catalysts for change by influencing and developing health policies and legislation that ban materials recognized as being related to a known disease or health condition.

Secondary prevention involves screening for diseases in a population, such as mammography and routine blood pressure measurements (CDC, 2019) and administering preventive drug therapies of proven effectiveness when given at an early stage of the disease (World Health Organization Eastern Mediterranean Regional Office [WHO EMRO], 2019). PHNs develop and coordinate screening programs, including educational content on the need for screening activities (WHO EMRO, 2019).

Tertiary prevention aims to reduce the impact of an ongoing illness or injury that may be long-term, is often complex, and has lasting effects. PHNs address tertiary prevention through educating and improving existing treatment modalities and potential recovery outcomes, including such activities as restoration and rehabilitation measures, medication management, and screenings for complications (CDC, 2019).

## 7. Ethics

Public health is committed to advancing the health and well-being of populations, not just individuals. Thus, one major challenge of public health ethics is providing an adequate analysis of what is morally at stake for individuals while maintaining its special connection to prevention for individuals and communities. Historically, public health ethics has drawn on multiple theories for its foundation. These theories include *deontology*, which focuses on duties and obligations to act, such as treating persons with respect because they have a moral status that makes them worthy of it. Another relevant theory is *utilitarianism*, with its goal of maximizing the greater good while preventing harm (Siegel & Merritt, 2019).

Many agree that the primary goal of public health should be ethical in nature (Beauchamp, 2003; Sherwin, 2008), and some view its moral foundation as justice (Faden et al., 2019). However, in recent years, many in public health have called for greater emphasis on social and environmental justice, equity, human rights, and well-being (Braveman, 2014; Braveman et al., 2011; LeClair et al., 2021; Powers & Faden, 2006; Srinivasan & Williams, 2014). Unfortunately, the continuing erosion of the public health infrastructure, along with the increasing recognition of the impact of poverty, health inequities, pandemics, systemic racism, violence, human rights violations, structural injustices, environmental crises, and disasters, have illustrated a need for such a shift in public health ethics (Brandt, 2021; Farmer, 2005; Powers & Faden, 2019; Watts et al., 2021).

Nursing focuses on protecting, promoting, and restoring health and abilities; preventing illness and injury; and alleviating suffering while caring for individuals, families, groups, communities, and populations. Nursing is broadly committed to the sick, injured, and vulnerable within society and to social and environmental justice (ANA, 2015a, 2015b). Over time, nursing ethics has gone from focusing on moral formation and virtue ethics to drawing on an ethics foundation focused on duties, obligations, relationships, consequences, and ethical principles (Fowler, 2020). Additionally, some nurses have studied in fields such as anthropology, education, philosophy, and ethics and have become familiar with critical social theory (Habermas, 1991), liberation theory (Freire, 1970, 1998), and feminist philosophy (Chodorow, 1978; Gilligan, 1982; Held, 2006; Noddings, 1984). Such diversity has contributed to the evolution of nursing, nursing ethics, and public health ethics.

Historically most recent nursing practice has been in hospitals and similar settings where the focus is primarily at the individual and family levels, with the application of ethics theories and principles in clinical situations focused on those levels. It is important to also remember that people live in the world and are embedded in multiple contexts and in diverse relationships with others. PH nursing identifies and intentionally bridges these contexts, emphasizing an ongoing commitment to populations, communities, and prevention as well as recognizing public health's concerns with social and environmental justice, equity, well-being, and health.

PHNs often face unique and difficult challenges that require understanding multiple ethical perspectives and frameworks as they bring together both public health and nursing. The history and events that occurred during the COVID-19 pandemic demonstrate how PH nursing will continue to face many complex challenges. At no previous time in the nation's past has the need for PHNs, and the need to study ethics, been greater.

# 8. Social Justice

Social justice is the moral foundation of public health, PH nursing, and health policy (Buettner-Schmidt & Lobo, 2011; Powers & Faden, 2006). Social justice efforts aspire to prevent injustices from occurring. The aims of social justice are well-being and health equity (Powers & Faden, 2006). Social justice is achieved by correcting institutional and structural conditions and factors that create injustices and inequalities and disadvantage or harm vulnerable groups (Young, 2011). Social justice includes the moral obligation to empower diverse, marginalized societal groups (Hagen et al., 2018). Social justice serves to support the concepts of "common" and "professional" morality (Lee & Zarowsky, 2015) in ensuring well-being and health equity through social structures and policies that promote access to opportunity and resources.

Powers and Faden (2006) introduced a theory of social justice that focuses on why justice matters in real-world concrete situations. They assert that a theory of justice should consider humans' well-being and how multiple determinants and their interrelatedness may influence this well-being along six essential dimensions that serve as a moral foundation for the social institution of public health: health, knowledge and understanding, personal security, equal respect, personal attachments, and self-determination. Powers and Faden contend that the focus of public policy development should be social justice and sufficiency in these dimensions to support the attainment of well-being essential to critical life stages, especially among the least advantaged or most vulnerable members of society. They propose that the application of an adequate theory of justice as fairness requires the use of empirical evidence as its justification (Powers & Faden, 2019). Critical evidence must reflect sufficient well-being across the life course in specific populations when developing, setting, and evaluating public policy and priorities for the just distribution of limited benefits and resources (Powers & Faden, 2006).

A persistent moral commitment to social justice is required of PHNs. This commitment includes an effort to collaborate with all stakeholders to promote the common good. PHNs are expected to pursue social justice and to be action-oriented and transformative to address the needs of diverse populations to move toward health equity across the nation (Sun, 2019; Thrift & Sugarman, 2019).

## 9. Health Equity

According to WHO, *health equity* is the absence of avoidable, unfair, or remediable differences among groups of people, whether those groups are defined socially, economically, demographically, geographically, or by other means of stratification (WHO, 2022). Health equity is achieved when every person has a fair opportunity to attain their full health potential and no one is disadvantaged from achieving this because of social position or other socially determined circumstances (CDC, n.d.-a). The Robert Wood Johnson Foundation provides a modified definition: "Health equity means that everyone has a fair and just opportunity to be as healthy as possible. This requires removing obstacles to health such as poverty, discrimination, and their consequences, including powerlessness and lack of access to good jobs with fair pay, quality education and housing, safe environments, and health care" (Braveman et al., 2017). The overall goal of public health is to maximize the health of the population, which means addressing health disparities and working toward health equity.

- Health equity has two core elements: (1) improving the health of those social groups who have historically been marginalized, excluded, or otherwise disadvantaged; and (2) not only improving health but modifying the SDOH (Braveman, 2019). Historically PHNs have focused on improving the human condition at all levels of community, particularly by reaching out to those most disadvantaged or marginalized. Working toward health equity and social and environmental justice is a core principle of PH nursing.

# THE ART AND SCIENCE OF PUBLIC HEALTH NURSING: A SYNERGY

PHNs promote the health of the public through the art and science of PH nursing practice, which is effectively the synergy of the practice of nursing and the practice of public health, as depicted in Figure 2.

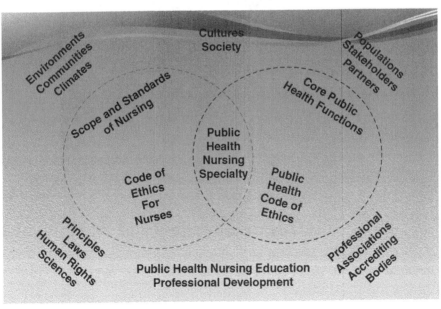

**Figure 2. The Dynamic Nature of Public Health Nursing (ANA, 2021)**

PH nursing uses an open and dynamic systems perspective along with a willingness to intentionally engage in interactions across systems with multiple stakeholders to promote the optimal health and well-being of populations and communities. The art of PH nursing means drawing on knowledge of nursing, social sciences, and public health science in combination with PH nursing experience. This is accomplished within the surrounding context of the social, built, and natural environments; populations, communities, climate, cultures, and society; stakeholders and partners; and educational and professional organizations. The PN nursing specialty acknowledges that people's contexts, knowledge, and lived experiences matter. This *Public Health Nursing: Scope & Standards of Practice, 3rd Edition* reflects both the nursing process and PH nursing practice competencies, as described in the Quad Council Coalition's (QCC) *Community/Public Health Nursing Competencies* (QCC Competency Review Task Force, 2018). Ethics, inherent to professional nursing, is expressed via the *Code of Ethics for Nurses with Interpretive Statements* (ANA, 2015a).

A variety of documents provides greater detail on elements of both public health and nursing practice that together outline key components of PH nursing practice. These include:

- The Core Functions of Public Health
- The Principles of Public Health Nursing Practice
- The 10 Essential Public Health Services
- The American Nurses Association's (ANA) *Public Health Nursing: Scope and Standards of Practice, Third Edition*, and the accompanying competencies
- The *Community/Public Health Nursing Competencies*, organized by eight practice domains (QCC Competency Review Task Force, 2018)

## CORE FUNCTIONS OF PUBLIC HEALTH

PH nursing practice involves application of the *core functions of public health*—assessment, policy development and assurance—which were originally defined to clarify the government's role in fulfilling the mission of public health (Institute of Medicine [IOM], 1988). PHNs integrate these core functions with the standards for PH nursing. Each core function is used in a systematic and comprehensive manner to achieve optimal health goals and is carried out in partnership with the public and other key stakeholders. As leaders in and advocates for these functions, PHNs are proactive on healthcare and social issues and build effective strategies to promote change:

- *Assessment* includes review of the concerns, strengths, and expectations of the population and is guided by epidemiological methods and the nursing process. Assessment uses both qualitative and quantitative data.
- *Policy development* is accomplished through the results of assessment, identification of the population's priorities, and consideration of other subpopulations and communities at greatest risk, using effective and evidence-based strategies. Policies may be developed within organizations and at all levels of government.
- *Assurance* is accomplished through regulation, advocacy for interdisciplinary services, coordination of community services, and (at times) direct provision of services. Assurance strategies consider the availability, acceptability, accessibility, effectiveness, and quality of services. (IOM, 1988)

## PRINCIPLES OF PUBLIC HEALTH NURSING PRACTICE

In 1997, the QCC of Public Health Nursing Organizations developed eight tenets or principles of PH nursing to advance the PH nursing goal of promoting and protecting the health of the population. The principles presented here have been adapted and refined to further describe the practice of PH nursing:

- *The primary focus of PH nursing practice is on systematic and comprehensive population-focused assessment, policy development, and assurance.*
  Although PHNs may engage in activities with individuals, families, groups, and at the system level, their dominant responsibility is to the population as a whole.
- *Equity is both a core public health value and a goal.*
  Equity is necessary to ensure optimal health and well-being for all. PHNs collaborate with members of other professions and

stakeholder groups to carry out the 10 Essential Services, which focus on achieving *equity*, defined as fairness.

- *Primary prevention is the priority in selecting appropriate activities.* Primary prevention includes health promotion as well as health protection and disease prevention strategies.
- *PH nursing focuses on strategies that create healthy social, environmental, and economic conditions in which populations may thrive.*
  PH nursing addresses SDOH through interventions that emerge from collaboration with the population. Advocacy and teaching advocacy skills to others are essential strategies when also addressing environmental and economic conditions.
- *PHNs collaborate with communities and populations as equal partners.* PHNs' actions must reflect awareness of the need for comprehensive health planning in partnership with communities and populations. Partnership includes understanding the perspectives, priorities, and values of the population when interpreting data, making policy and program decisions, and selecting appropriate strategies for action.
- *Collaboration with members of other professions, organizations, and stakeholder groups as well as the population is the most effective way to promote and protect the health and well-being of the community.* Creating the conditions for optimizing health and well-being is an extremely complex, resource-intensive process. To create these conditions, PHNs join others from a variety of fields and professions and partner with community members who are local experts. Leadership in this effort recognizes the importance of involvement in the health care system, legislative action, and social policy agendas.
- *PHNs are obligated to actively identify and reach out to all who might benefit from a specific activity or service.*
  Specific subpopulations may be marginalized and more vulnerable to preventable disease, illness, and death, often having more difficulty in accessing or using the available services. Vulnerable populations require special outreach efforts beyond those efforts directed at the general population. PHNs focus on the whole population and not just those who present for services.

- *Optimal use of available resources and creation of new evidence-based public health strategies are necessary to enhance the health of the population.*

Resource use and strategy creation include:

o Organizing and coordinating action responses to health issues;

o Using and providing to decision makers evidence-based public health and cost-effectiveness information related to outcomes of specific actions, programs, or policies; and

o Researching and designing the collection of evidence as the foundation for the practice of population-based care.

## THE 10 ESSENTIAL PUBLIC HEALTH SERVICES

In 1994, a Centers for Disease Control and Prevention (CDC) steering committee, comprising representatives from US public health service agencies and other major public health organizations, developed a set of 10 essential services to provide a working operationalization of the core functions of public health. These 10 Essential Public Health Services are a guiding framework for the responsibilities of community public health systems. These services were reviewed and revised in 2020 (CDC, 2020, March 18). Public health systems are to undertake the following public health activities (CDC, 2020, March 18):

1. Assess and monitor population health status, factors that influence health, and community needs and assets.
2. Investigate, diagnose, and address health problems and hazards affecting the population.
3. Communicate effectively to inform and educate people about health, factors that influence it, and how to improve it.
4. Strengthen, support, and mobilize communities and partnerships to improve health.
5. Create, champion, and implement policies, plans, and laws that impact health.
6. Utilize legal and regulatory actions designed to improve and protect the public's health.
7. Ensure an effective system that enables equitable access to the individual services and care needed to be healthy.

8. Build and support a diverse and skilled public health workforce.
9. Improve and innovate public health functions through ongoing evaluation, research, and continuous quality improvement.
10. Build and maintain a strong organizational infrastructure for public health.

Additionally, ethics is inherent to public health and is exemplified in the *Public Health Code of Ethics* (APHA, 2019).

Figure 3 illustrates the synergy of the 10 Essential Services of Public Health and the Principles of Public Health Nursing Practice, resulting in a rich overlap of public health philosophy that forms the basis for PHNs' practice (Public Health Nursing Standards of Practice).

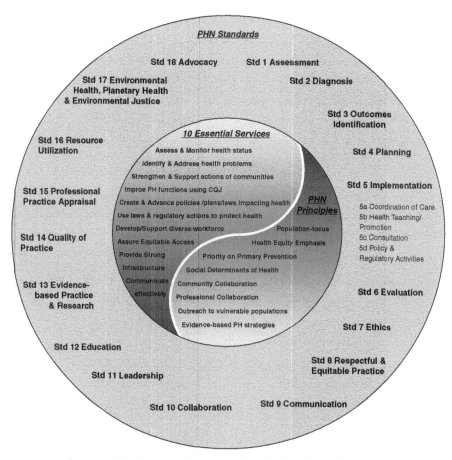

**Figure 3. The Synergy Between Public Health and Nursing**

# Public Health Nursing Standards and Competencies

### 1. Public Health Nursing Standards of Practice

The complete set of PH nursing standards of practice and professional performance and the accompanying competencies on pages xxxx are congruent with the template language of *Nursing: Scope and Standards of Practice, Third Edition* (ANA, 2015b). The crosswalk analysis of these standards with the Community/Public Health Nursing Competencies (QCC Competency Review Task Force, 2018) identifies coherence and consistency between the two sets.

### 2. Community/Public Health Nursing Competencies

The Council of Public Health Nursing Organizations (formerly the QCC of Public Health Nursing organizations) developed *The Community/Public Health Nursing Competencies* (QCC Competency Review Task Force, 2018), organized by eight public health domains, as defined by the Council on Linkages (CoL; 2017):

- Analytic Assessment;
- Policy Development/Program Planning;
- Communication;
- Cultural Competency;
- Community Dimensions of Practice;
- Basic Public Health Sciences;
- Financial Planning and Management; and
- Leadership and Systems Thinking.

The accompanying practice competencies for each domain were divided into three tiers to reflect PH nursing:

- Tier 1 is competencies for PHNs.
- Tier 2 is for PHNs practicing at an advanced PH nursing practice level.
- Tier 3 is for those advanced public health nurses (APHNs) in executive leadership positions.

All tiers address the Core Functions of Public Health—(1) Assessment, (2) Policy Development, and (3) Assurance (CDC, 2011)—as well as the 10 Essential Services (CDC, 2020, March 18).

# Roles and Functions of Public Health Nurses

Previous sections have described the definition of PH nursing practice, its foundations, and its context. This section provides an overview of **how** PHNs practice, including relevant roles and functions.

### PUBLIC HEALTH 3.0 AND CULTURE OF HEALTH

Public health has evolved over time, moving from the early traditions of *Public Health 1*, focused on sanitation, food and water safety, and tracking communicable diseases as an emerging government responsibility, to *Public Health 2.0*, with public health services developing into disease-specific programs (DeSalvo et al., 2017). Current public health practice is moving into version 3.0, in which practitioners of public health work across sectors and disciplines to address SDOH and improve community health broadly (DeSalvo et al., 2017). Traditionally, PHNs have worked in public health programs promoting health and preventing disease across specific targeted populations. However, community health promotion efforts that have addressed health inequities and SDOH have always been an integral part of PHNs' practice. Hence, the move to *Public Health 3.0* is a natural evolution for PH nursing practice, using the nursing process and community engagement (CE) for broad, cross disciplinary, and intersectoral health promotion efforts.

The Robert Wood Johnson Foundation proclaimed a need to advance a Culture of Health in 2013 (Chandra et al., 2017). Such a culture places well-being at the center of every aspect of life, with the overall goal of enabling everyone to lead healthier lives. The Action Framework for developing this Culture of Health includes four elements: making health a shared value; fostering cross-sector collaboration to improve well-being; creating healthier, more equitable communities; and strengthening integration of health services and systems. These four elements align well with both *Public Health 3.0* and the roles of PHNs in engaging communities, building cross-sector collaboration, and leveraging their health care system and public health knowledge to engage and provide leadership. PHNs continue to embrace the provision of services to individuals and families. However, the overall focus of PH nursing practice is on what benefits the total population, such as addressing SDOH and advancing health equity.

## HEALTH PROMOTION AND PROTECTION

Multi-drug-resistant organisms; bioterrorism events; lack of access to SDOH, such as food and safe housing; and anti-vaccination campaigns have increased the risk of disease in communities. An increase in the number of families in which all adults work outside the home leads to more families accessing childcare, with resultant increased exposure to infectious diseases at an early age. Partnerships with health care providers to promote antibiotic stewardship through education campaigns and support for vaccinations in all settings are protection strategies employed by PHNs in the community. Collaboration with food banks, schools, landlords, and childcare centers to encourage handwashing, respiratory hygiene, exercise, healthy eating, and traffic safety are activities that promote healthy behaviors and can be encouraged with PH nursing support.

---

### HEALTH PROMOTION & PROTECTION

"Creating a Healthy Community" was a community engagement day organized by local PHNs in partnership with community-based organizations. The local health department, local businesses, major employers, health care organizations, mental health organizations, and churches planned the event to address community health needs identified in the county's Community Health Needs Assessment.

In addition to serving as community organizers during the planning phase, PHNs oversaw blood pressure, weight, and happiness/stress screenings during the event. Several PHNs led group coaching sessions to help participants set SMART (specific, measurable, attainable, realistic, and timebound) personal health and well-being goals. As part of the group coaching sessions, participants identified the first steps they will take toward reaching each of their goals, how to identify an "accountability buddy" to check in with as they work toward their goals, and how they will celebrate reaching milestones in their health and well-being journey.

---

Planetary health problems, such as climate change, global migration, stressors of war, and a shortage of essential resources, are making it increasingly difficult for vulnerable populations to achieve a sense of well-being and good health, especially in times of disaster. With an emphasis on primary prevention, PHNs promote community resilience by emphasizing preparedness activities (such as sharing natural disaster risk assessments, stockpiling necessities, establishing evacuation routes, etc.) to plan for the impact of disruptive events.

---

### EMERGENCY PREPAREDNESS & DISASTER RECOVERY

When the pandemic struck and PHNs were assigned to the Operations Section/Vaccination Distribution Branch, everyone remembered why the Federal Emergency Management Agency (FEMA) trainings on emergency response had been required. Mass vaccinations clinics were initiated.

As PHNs oversaw mass vaccination clinics, data were showing that the community's most vulnerable populations were not being reached. A group of communicable disease PHNs devised a plan for outreach activities to the communities where members of the vulnerable populations eat, sleep, play, and pray. One PHN volunteered to work with the local homeless shelter to engage that population in discussions around vaccine hesitancy. Another visited a home for women and children to educate about the benefits of vaccines. And a small team organized a vaccine clinic at a local mall. Vaccine rates in the vulnerable populations increased, and disease rates decreased dramatically after PHNs launched these initiatives.

---

PHNs serve on the front lines and behind the scenes in the event of an emergency or disaster, assisting in the alleviation of immediate needs, such as access to clean water, safe food, and disease prevention. In this role, PHNs partner with disaster relief agencies, housing authorities, and environmental health professionals. PHNs may assist in family reunification efforts and use their nursing skills to help communities in crisis stabilize families until mental health resources are available.

In the recovery phase, PHNs are instrumental in assisting response agencies to identify those who are most vulnerable, locate resources within a community, and mobilize the community. These partnerships with various agencies may include offering local shelter services where nursing resources are scarce or setting up vaccination clinic points of distribution to provide needed immunizations. PHNs assist in the development of systems to mitigate the impact of future events by partnering with health care providers, emergency management services (EMS), and others to lead advocacy efforts for vulnerable populations and help identify where resources are needed.

One recent example of the role of PHNs has been in response to the COVID-19 Pandemic. This pandemic has threatened lives and exacerbated existing health inequities. PHNs have worked in the pandemic across all sectors to coordinate and facilitate prevention, testing, immunization and other interventions and have assisted in the development of policies locally, nationally, and globally.

## ENVIRONMENTAL SAFETY AND QUALITY

PHNs often collaborate with their environmental health colleagues to assess and mitigate exposures that can affect a community. Such collaboration may happen at the individual level, by referring a child with an elevated blood-lead level, or at the community level when citizens are encountering unsafe levels of contaminants in drinking water. Assessing the health impacts of a physically unsafe environment (e.g., domestic violence or unsafe playgrounds) on a child's development is part of the PH nursing scope of practice. Furthermore, PHNs seek to promote healthy sustainable environments that provide clean water, air, land, food, and energy as well as products free of known toxins. Such assessments may identify work- and community-related exposures to pesticides, fertilizers, weed control, and other agents for vulnerable workers, such as orchard, vineyard, and farm workers. PHNs assess the quality of the available evidence in determining whether the environmental issue being addressed is local, state, or national and requires advocacy, policy, public education, or other interventions. PHNs recognize that climate change is an ongoing public health concern that requires associated advocacy and public education.

## ENVIRONMENTAL SAFETY & QUALITY

Maternal/infant PHN specialists, as part of the Postpartum/Newborn Home Visiting Program, began to be concerned about their patients and families living in older, substandard housing. Armed with lead-testing swabs, PHNs launched "No Lead in My Bed," a small community health program to find environmental sources of lead in homes.

The program resulted in the discovery of lead paint in some of the older homes. Old plastic blinds, imported years ago and known to contain lead, were common and often found hanging above infants' cribs. One home had an old kitchen cabinet with flaking paint above the counter where the new mother was preparing her baby's formula.

PHNs reached out to a local abatement business that had received special funding for renovations in low-income residences and routinely conducted lead testing prior to initiating their renovation work. However, company policy prevented lead abatement in houses with renters who might soon move out. PHNs reminded the company managers that there was a very good chance that another low-income family would shortly take this family's place. The PHNs used advocacy, education, and innovation to make safer homes for families and newborns.

### CLINICAL INTERVENTIONS

PHNs may employ clinical care strategies, such as direct observed therapy for active tuberculosis cases, immunizations for vulnerable groups, prophylaxis for contacts to those exposed to communicable diseases, and quarantine/isolation activities. In line with public health practice, these clinical interventions are directed at protecting the entire population. The Minnesota Intervention Wheel, previously discussed, illustrates the public health interventions applicable for PH nursing practice, including screening, case finding, case management, and delegated functions of direct care services (Minnesota Department of Health, 2019).

## CARE COORDINATION

Care coordination involves deliberately organizing the care activities of individuals and sharing information among all the participants concerned with that care. The goal is to achieve safer and more effective care. This means that the individual's needs and preferences are known ahead of time and communicated at the right time to the right people and that this information is used to provide safe, appropriate, and effective care to individuals and groups (Agency for Healthcare Research and Quality [AHRQ], 2014). For PH nursing practice, this involves coordination of care within and across the continuum, including community agencies and schools, addressing social needs for individuals and families and SDOH at the community and policy levels. In addition, the PHN role can include advocating for access to needed services for an individual or community to maximize health.

---

### CARE COORDINATION

The PHN met with a young family with a child with special needs who had recently moved to the area. The PHN's comprehensive assessment included the child's clinical, psychosocial, and social needs; the parent's social and financial needs; the family's history of experiences with governmental and community support; the family's and child's strengths, concerns, and desires; and the child's specific care activities and needs. The PHN led the creation of an interprofessional care coordination team and comprehensive plan of care to address clinical and social milestones.

The PHN also supported the family as they set goals regarding childcare so the parents could go to work. Assessment of community resources identified organizations that help kids with special needs develop friendships and stay social. The PHN continued to advocate and coordinate care for the child and family by interacting with the government, condition-specific associations, and community connections. The child received the required care.

---

## CROSS-SECTOR COLLABORATION; COMMUNITY ENGAGEMENT/PARTNERSHIPS

Community engagement (CE) is an essential strategy for PHNs who are working with communities. CE has been defined by the CDC (2011) as "the process of working collaboratively with groups of people who are affiliated by geographic proximity, special interests or similar situations with respect to issues affecting their well-being." CE is a process extending from reaching out to community members (outreach) to consulting with them (consultation) to partner to develop shared goals and implement activities to address community needs (collaboration). This collaborative approach emphasizes mutuality, whereby community partners identify and prioritize what needs are to be addressed. CE involves trust building and facilitating equity when implementing community-based interventions (CDC, 2011).

---

### COLLABORATION & PARTNERSHIP

A local Black community was experiencing a high HIV infection rate. Because many successful social-change efforts within communities of color historically have been led by faith organizations, the PHN decided to begin addressing this issue by first approaching the local Black church. The PHN met with the pastor and the church council to discuss increasing rates of HIV in their community and to explore collaborative efforts to educate the community about HIV and connect them with resources to help them lead healthier lives.

Through education and engagement, the PHN was able to get buy-in from the faith-based leaders, which opened the door to engaging the community members. Together, they planned an evening meeting with a favorite meal, where the PHN provided a low-key presentation on the high rates of HIV in the community. The PHN established trust with the community members because he answered their questions with facts and without judgment. That initiative grew steadily. Eventually, increased rates of HIV testing led to increased rates of treatment and a remarkable decrease in the number of new HIV diagnoses. This initial partnership led to other health promotion activities in the community, including basic school health screenings and screenings for hypertension and diabetes.

---

*Community-Based Participatory Research*—Community-based participatory research (CBPR) focuses on establishing equitable partnerships, addressing a population's needs based in collaboration with them, and responding to what the community has identified as the primary issue. Competence in CBPR is a core requirement for specialists in public health (PHF, 2014) and PH nursing (QCC Competency Review Task Force, 2018). Public health professionals contribute scientific evidence by participating in CBPR (PHF, 2014) and other "research activities impacting the health of populations" (QCC Competency Review Task Force, 2018, p. 25). All PHNs engaging in and leading CBPR must understand what is at stake for communities and populations. CBPR raises concern for the ethical treatment of groups, incorporates an obligation to take community views into account, and protects vulnerable communities from harm because ethical issues can arise during research (Guba & Lincoln, 1989).

## RESEARCH

An APHN became concerned upon discovering an increased number of post-menopausal women treated for sexually transmitted infections (STI) and convinced state leaders to fund a local university research program to determine STI incidence, prevalence, and disease outbreak trends in women between 55 and 75 years old. Concurrently, the APHN conducted a research program to further explore demographics; history of STI; health behaviors ranging from nutrition, sleep habits, and physical and sexual activity; and knowledge of healthy sexual behaviors in women of the same age group. Using the findings from both studies, the APHN advocated to the legislature for increased state funding for sexual health programs, resulting in approval of an 80% increase in program funding.

Mutuality is a core principle that guides CBPR, suggesting that all parties contribute equitably and benefit from an interdependent relationship. Implementing mutuality requires respect for persons as autonomous, self-determining, and also connected and embedded within contexts and relationships (Wallwork, 2008). Demonstrating and maintaining respect for persons whose views differ make fostering dialogue, establishing trust, and developing collaborative relations essential to CBPR (Baldwin et al., 2009; Wallwork, 2008). CBPR is complex, challenging, and takes time. CBPR researchers need to be open, flexible, able to live with uncertainty, and trusting of dynamic processes (Edwards et al., 2008).

*Epidemiological Research*—Epidemiological methods are employed to determine sources of a disease outbreak, the incidence or prevalence of an existing disease, the natural history of a disease, and risk factors for a disease within a population or community. These epidemiologic research processes then lead to mobilizing interventions to mitigate the problem. Given that epidemiology includes surveillance of disease trends, PHNs use data to monitor these trends and inform further data collection. In leadership levels, PHNs strategically collaborate with civic leaders, tribal councils, or other groups to identify possible unintended consequences of the use of data, such as stigma or lack of culturally appropriate interventions.

## POLICY AND ADVOCACY

Policy development is a core function of public health and a required competency for all public health professionals and PHNs (PHF, 2014; PHLS, 2002). In addition, developing health policies is one of the standards required for public health agency accreditation (2015). When determining public health priorities, SDOH, health risks, and poor health outcomes of specific populations are to be considered. New or revised policies must address alleviating causes of health inequity. Such changes can address social, economic, and environmental conditions that affect "health equity, including housing, transportation, education, job availability, neighborhood safety, and zoning" (Public Health Accreditation Board [PHAB], 2014, p. 5).

Advocacy for individuals, families, populations, and communities is one of the standards of PH nursing practice (Standard 18). PHNs must speak for the communities and population and participate in the legislative process, reflecting the expectation of all public health professionals to engage in "advocacy for policies, programs, and resources that improve health in a community (e.g., using evidence to demonstrate the need for a program, communicating the impact of a program)" (PHF, 2014, p. 16).

## Distinguishing Public Health Nursing from Other Nursing Specialties

As a specialty grounded in both nursing and public health sciences, PH nursing focuses on population health skills at the community and systems end of the ecological model. Examples of population-focused care include a focus on laws, regulations, organizations, systems, programs, and policies by working with key stakeholders to influence health and social conditions to optimize a population's health.

Another distinguishing characteristic of PH nursing practice is the goal of improving a population's health with an emphasis on health promotion, disease prevention, and risk reduction. Thus, the setting is not the defining characteristic of PH nursing. Although not all PHNs work in community settings, partnering with populations in communities is the cornerstone of PH nursing practice.

### APPLICATION OF THE NURSING PROCESS IN PUBLIC HEALTH NURSING

The nursing process is "a systematic approach to care using the fundamental principles of critical thinking, client-centered approaches to treatment, goal-oriented tasks, evidence-based practice recommendations, and nursing intuition" (Toney-Butler & Thayer, 2020). All professional nurses use the nursing process. However, in this nursing specialty, application of PH nursing principles guides decision-making in each step of the nursing process (Alexander, 2020).

Through the nursing process's systematic application, PHNs assess health status, identify issues/needs/problems/assets, develop a plan and identify relevant outcome indicators based on the best available evidence and priorities, implement the plan, and evaluate the outcomes at the systems, community, population, group, family, and individual levels. The steps are carried out in partnership with the systems, organizations, and members of the community/population of interest.

Below is an outline of how the PH nursing process is carried out when working with a population (Alexander, 2020; Center for Public Health Nursing Practice, 2003).

### Assessment

When working with a population, the first step of the PH nursing process includes identifying and clarifying the population of interest. PHNs reach out and establish a mutual relationship of trust with members of the population and open dialogue to further refine the issues/needs/problems.

PHNs also engage partnering organizations with a stake in the population's health and the issue/need/problem that could be involved in the intervention. PHNs guide the assessment process, incorporating the population's and stakeholder's observations and insights specific to the issue, which are key to a comprehensive and correct assessment.

## Diagnosis

PHNs use clinical judgment to identify possible diagnoses that will be the basis for the care plan specific to the population's identified issue/need/problem. PHNs communicate with members of the population and key stakeholders to reach a consensus diagnosis that reflects their perception of the issue/need/problem and the desired changes.

## Plan

In the planning step, PHNs collaborate with the population and stakeholder organizations to set goals and select health status outcome indicators specific to the issue/need/problem. PHNs ensure that the population's input is an essential component in selecting evidence-based or innovative best-practice interventions that will resonate with the population, increase participation in the intervention, and identify appropriate evaluation methods for the intervention population. PHNs identify any barriers to implementation and advocate for resources to break down those barriers.

## Implementation

During the implementation step, PHNs communicate with members of the population who are participating in the intervention and stakeholder organizations involved in its implementation. PHNs provide ongoing guidance to address issues that arise, promote facts, answer questions, and encourage participation in the intervention.

## Evaluation

PHNs work with the population and stakeholders to determine the plan's and intervention's effectiveness through ongoing collection and comparison of evaluation data to the overall goal and objectives. PHNs communicate with the population and involved stakeholders if the plan or intervention must be modified to achieve the goal and objectives. PHNs communicate the intervention results to members of the population, public health colleagues, and other key stakeholders. PHNs encourage systems modifications as appropriate to help sustain changes.

PHNs' unique contributions bring the nursing process into public health work in all settings. Such action ensures that colleagues, populations, community members, groups, families, and individuals are equal partners throughout the PH nursing process.

### COLLABORATING AND BUILDING PARTNERSHIPS

By recognizing the important linkages and relationships within a community, PHNs acknowledge the need to organize their interventions within a framework that addresses the connections between the population and the environment. All professional nurses collaborate with other health and social service professionals, but PHNs collaborate and build partnerships with individuals, families, communities, other professions, and systems of care (Pittman, 2019).

Interprofessional collaboration and participation on interdisciplinary teams is a strategy that PHNs use to achieve public health goals. Additionally, PHNs collaborate across sectors of the community, such as transportation, recreation, and economics, to promote public health (Anderson & McFarlane, 2019). Ample evidence supports interprofessional work and community-based solutions as effective approaches to increasing health equity (NASEM, 2017). Building partnerships within and outside the health sector and leveraging these relationships allow for collaborative solutions to improve the health of individuals, families, and communities (Pittman, 2019).

### POLICY DEVELOPMENT AND IMPLEMENTATION

PHNs engage in policy development and implementation as an essential part of their practice that advances the health of the public. PHNs must be attuned to changes in health, economic, and social policies that affect populations at the local, state, federal, and international levels. Involvement in developing and monitoring strategies related to current or future health care laws and regulations is an important contribution to promoting and protecting the health of the public. Ensuring that health and economic policy content is integrated into all levels of PH nursing education and practice is equally important.

Continued shifts in health policy and evolving models of health care delivery and reimbursement require ongoing monitoring to understand their influence on public health outcomes. Emergence of accountable care organizations and value-based purchasing are examples of models that may affect the public's health. PHNs evaluate the outcomes of community- and population-level interventions to fully articulate the return on investment (ROI). Assessing ROI is especially important as local, state, federal, and international budgets related to the provision of health care services shrink and public scrutiny increases.

## PROMOTING SOCIAL AND ENVIRONMENTAL JUSTICE AND ETHICAL DECISION-MAKING

PHNs must recognize and establish their professional practice in accordance with the population's rights and with concern for social and environmental justice. Identifying and advocating for upstream solutions is an essential strategy when confronting systemic injustices (Pittman, 2019). In addition, the precautionary principle guides decision-making and acknowledges that, in the absence of sufficient scientific evidence, the appropriate action is caution and avoidance of unnecessary risk. PHNs explore alternatives to potentially harmful actions as well as promote increased public participation in decision-making (Chaudry, 2008). In addition, PHNs must ensure that ethical issues are addressed as part of the decision-making process and should also be competent to serve on ethics bodies that make decisions affecting the rights of the populations they serve.

Advocacy focused on public health is another important facet of PH nursing. PHNs inform and educate populations to enhance their self-care and address SDOH and access to health care. PHNs advocate on behalf of marginalized populations for safe housing, environmental justice, access to food, and access to health care delivered in an equitable, fair, and competent manner, regardless of health insurance status or the presence of illness or disease.

According to the US Census Bureau (2015), by 2044, the majority of the US population will be composed of traditionally underrepresented ethnic minorities. These changing demographics call for PHNs to have an increased awareness of barriers to health care for all populations. PHNs need to recognize the important influence that culture plays in overall health. In addition, PHNs should acknowledge the diverse cultural backgrounds represented within the populations they serve. PHNs must practice cultural safety and be able to effectively communicate with people in the communities with whom they work. PHNs must also acknowledge their own cultural lens, which affects their ability to integrate cultural humility into their nursing practice.

Ethics is a complex area. However, many ethics theories, concepts, definitions, relationships, underlying beliefs, and guiding principles can be practically applicable and useful in decision-making when facing real-world situations and challenges (Summers, 2014). Such situations can be complex and fraught with uncertainty and ambiguity; they may have no one solution or no guarantee of a correct solution, and even experts may disagree about what actions to take to address them (Churchman, 1971). PHNs frequently face situations that pose ethical challenges, dilemmas, or conflicts, whatever their role, the practice setting, or the focus of their practice (individuals, families, communities, or populations). When such situations arise, they require careful consideration, ethical analysis, and decision-making.

One approach to decision-making involves applying knowledge of ethics theories and principles while engaging in a reasoning process to arrive at a solution. Rawls (1971) refers to this process as "reflective equilibrium," where one considers the situation from multiple perspectives or viewpoints, considers competing ethics theories or principles, and considers conflicting moral claims. A moral claim is what is at stake in the situation and for whom; such claims can conflict. PHNs are frequently called upon to make decisions in the face of ethical uncertainty about correct decisions and uncertain knowledge of the outcomes (Summers, 2014). PHNs may be called upon to explain their reasons for such decisions so that appropriate, and at times morally urgent, actions can be taken.

PHNs do not practice in isolation and are encouraged to engage in discussions with appropriate colleagues and stakeholders in their efforts to understand, analyze, and respond appropriately to ethical challenges. Depending on the setting, an ethics consultant may be available to meet with PHNs and to participate in discussions while providing information and support. Currently, ethics committees are more common in large institutions and agencies (Farber Post & Blustein, 2015; Hester & Schonfeld, 2016), and depending on the agency and jurisdiction, they may only meet once a month.

Ethics committees often have a specific responsibility and are comprised of agency and community members with appropriate backgrounds. It is important for ethics committee members to be familiar with federal and state laws, as these may influence ethical decisions (Latham, 2016). Some agencies, such as state health departments, may only have institutional review committees that focus on public health research, although individual counties and tribal nations may establish ethics committees to help address community- and population-level concerns.

Because their specialty bridges the domains of public health and nursing, PHNs are expected to be familiar with two formal *codes of ethics: Code of Ethics for Nurses with Interpretive Statements* (ANA, 2015a) and *Public Health Code of Ethics* (APHA, 2019). These codes provide guidance for action and include inspirational and aspirational ideals, but they are not laws and do not provide all the answers to ethical questions. PHNs must be able to analyze the situations occurring in practice and appropriately apply the guidelines in particular situations.

Codes of ethics are supported by various theories and approaches to ethics, many of which have already been mentioned. For example, care ethics focuses on relations, acknowledging persons as interdependent and as simultaneously embedded in multiple contexts, such as family and community (Carse, 1996; Chodorow, 1978; Gilligan, 1982; Held, 2006; Noddings, 1984). Care ethics attends to context, emotions, lived experiences, narrative, mutual vulnerability, identity, connection, and the concrete, particular self in relation. Care ethics focuses on meeting the needs of others, broadened beyond individuals to include communities and populations, for whom one has responsibility during times of vulnerability and is practically applicable in real-world contexts.

PHNs and APHNs are expected to integrate the provisions of the 2015 Code of Ethics for *Nurses with Interpretive Statements* in their practice. The examples accompanying each of the provisions are intended to help provide understanding of an application of the provision in PH nursing practice.

**Provision 1. *The nurse practices with compassion and respect for the inherent dignity, worth, and unique attributes of every person.***

A nursing faculty member accompanied PHN students to the downtown area of a major city in an innovative approach to help students conduct community assessments, identify community needs, and learn about the value of community outreach to anyone who might need assistance. They started the day by partnering with members of a local church, including the parish priest, parish nurse, and a social worker at an outreach center serving this diverse urban community. The outreach center offers community members, persons without housing or experiencing unstable housing, and older adults living in nearby apartments a safe place to gather, seek assistance, and address shared community challenges, such as limited access to fresh foods, clothing, and shelter.

On that first day of clinical, the nursing students completed two guided tours of the community, led by outreach center volunteers who were also community members. One volunteer, having experienced homelessness, focused their tour on what a day is like spent searching for food, drinking water, restroom facilities, and shelter while continuously walking to avoid being assaulted, harassed, or arrested. Another volunteer took the students to a cramped neighborhood grocery that mainly offered canned fruits, vegetables, soups, and meats high in sodium with limited fresh vegetables, minimal healthy food, and over-the-counter medication choices.

The PHN students were able to experience firsthand the importance of respect for the dignity and rights of all human beings, regardless of their circumstances or factors contributing to their health. By observing the outreach center's volunteers and staff interacting with the community members, and the community members' response to being treated with courtesy, civility, and integrity, the PHN students also learned that a person's worth is not affected by illness, ability, socioeconomic status, or other factors. This deeper understanding enabled the PHN students to practice their compassion and respect for those they served throughout their month-long community rotation.

*Provision 2. The nurse's primary commitment is to the patient, whether an individual, family, group, community, or population.*

As the COVID-19 pandemic expanded across the state, local efforts to promote the health and well-being of community members were severely curtailed, and the local outreach center needed to close. The community faced new challenges, such as finding housing and other basic resources for those without reliable shelter. Community members without homes needed a room or apartment where they could socially distance themselves from ill persons, or even isolate themselves if they became ill with COVID-19. They also needed delivery of food, medications, sheets, blankets, clothing, face masks, soap or hand sanitizer, and other items, along with periodic visits to help monitor and promote their recovery or to access other levels of care.

The local health department's PHN administrator wanted to help and approached the health director about the community's needs, but they were told to direct all energy toward COVID-19 and the mass vaccine and testing efforts and that the community would take care of its own. The PHN administrator understood that the mass vaccination and testing efforts were the top priority of the state's Board of Health but also knew that the community members facing diminishing resources during a pandemic could not be pushed aside. The PHN developed a proposal suggesting that the already trained assistant PHN administrator take over the management of the mass vaccine and testing efforts for two weeks so the PHN administrator could collaborate with local businesses on how to best meet the needs of the vulnerable community. The proposal presentation to the health director emphasized that the needs of both populations could be met. After some negotiation, the PHN administrator was able to redirect efforts to help the community members displaced by the closing of the outreach center.

***Provision 3. The nurse promotes, advocates for, and protects the rights, health, and safety of the patient.***

During the final day of a public health clinical rotation, a diverse group of nursing students who were graduating the following spring gathered to watch *Sentimental Women Need Not Apply: A History of the American Nurse* (Garey & Hott,1988). The film included a clip about the history of PH nursing. The African American students in the group wondered aloud why no one had ever shown them the film before.

They listened carefully to nurses voicing their views and describing their nursing experiences. The students' sense of pride began to swell as an African American nurse historian began to speak about Mary Mahoney, the first Black professionally trained nurse to graduate in the United States. They heard that Black nurses had volunteered to serve during WWII. The students spoke openly and with excitement about what they were hearing and confirmed this was the first time they felt like they belonged in nursing. They believed that this part of nursing history was missing from their nursing education. Whatever the reasons for its absence or omission, the students were now paying close attention to this history that they were joining.

The students had just spent the semester in a PH nursing rotation, working with predominantly African Americans living in poverty, in unstable or unsafe housing, or even without housing. By working with the community, the students had come to understand the very important contributions they could make to the nursing profession by enhancing its diversity, promoting health and well-being in their own communities, and advocating for and protecting the people living there. The students' experiences had salience and value and stood out for them as exemplars.

***Provision 4. The nurse has authority, accountability, and responsibility for nursing practice; makes decisions; and takes action consistent with the obligation to promote health and to provide optimal care.***

During a weekly home visit to see a two-year-old child and her mother, a PHN finds bruises on the child's back. The PHN carefully discusses her concerns with the mother, who admits that the baby's father lost his temper and hit the child the day before. The PHN completes a social assessment and a domestic violence screening and then tells the mom that she will need to report her findings to child protection services. She also tells the mother that she will continue to support her and the child with their weekly home visits and offers to help the mother get support to relocate, if she is ready. The PHN shares with the mother the steps that she will take in following her agency's protocols and state law for mandatory reporting and calls in the initial report with the mother and child by her side. Before leaving, the PHN verifies once again that the mother is still not ready to go to a safer environment and reinforces her willingness to help at any time, should she change her mind.

*Provision 5. The nurse owes the same duties to self as to others, including the responsibility to promote health and safety, preserve wholeness of character and integrity, maintain competence, and continue personal and professional growth.*

The COVID-19 pandemic has presented a great challenge in that many nurses have been witnesses to the devastation resulting from the virus. Nurses have been encouraged to obtain the COVID-19 vaccine to protect themselves, their clients, families, friends, and co-workers. Many nurses expressed relief when the vaccine became available and celebrated the opportunity to receive it and protect themselves and others while preventing the virus's spread.

A PHN was struggling with the decision about whether he should get the COVID-19 vaccine. His wife, mother, father, and in-laws were strongly opposed to the vaccine for religious reasons and were leaning heavily on him to not receive it. The PHN was experiencing moral distress because he struggled to balance his values related to his religion, which were very important to him, and his values as a nurse, which were grounded in his belief in the science behind the vaccines. The PHN decided to have a family conference and talk to them about his concerns and moral distress. He explained to them how important his religion and his family's wishes were to him. He reminded them of why he initially had chosen to go to nursing school and shared why he had later chosen to specialize in public health. He then explained that because he believed in the science of public health and the benevolence of receiving the vaccine when others could not, he had decided that he would get it. His family realized that his values were aligned and voiced their support of his decision.

*Provision 6. The nurse, through individual and collective effort, establishes, maintains, and improves the ethical environment of the work setting and conditions of employment that are conducive to safe, quality health care.*

When establishing a new community health center, the clinic's charge nurse engaged with the clinic's leader and other health care team members to help them establish and implement the center's core values, which included mission, vision, and value statements. Once the community health center opened, this nurse reinforced this effort by placing placards displaying the core values throughout the clinic and discussing them during clinic staff meetings. The clinic's charge nurse also orchestrated the dissemination via placement of the core values on the clinic's fliers, letterhead, website, and personnel email signature lines. The charge nurse demonstrated the core values on a continual basis and created a safe place for open communication and dialogue among personnel throughout the workday and outside work settings. This nurse reinforced the core values by regularly giving positive feedback to the health care team members who demonstrated positive, ethical behavior among each other and with clients. The clinic's charge nurse also partnered with vendors that had the same core values as the clinic.

*Provision 7. The nurse, in all roles and settings, advances the profession through research and scholarly inquiry, professional standards development, and the generation of both nursing and health policy.*

A PHN was invited to consult with a county health department's maternal and child health program to work on a project related to the use of community health workers (CHW) with women at high risk for poor pregnancy outcomes. The PHN invited key stakeholders, including local PHNs, CHWs, and several women of child-bearing age living in the surrounding area, to participate in planning the project. The PHN consultant facilitated the group's dialogue, decision-making process, planning, and implementation of a comprehensive community and population assessment, which included a formal research component.

Together, the group developed questions and modified a standardized tool to assess what social support was available and used by local women at high risk for poor pregnancy outcomes. The group also created an agency marketing survey to determine whether and which local agencies had similar concerns. The comprehensive assessment included a review of relevant literature and research, a review of local data and information over time, a review of organizational structures and processes, and a review of health policies that may influence what services were available, their funding sources, who was eligible for services, and how one obtained such services.

After receiving Institutional Review Board approval of the research component prior to its implementation, the PHN consultant educated the local PHNs on how to oversee the project research and data analysis activities. The CHWs were trained to assist in conducting research interviews, surveys, and data collection. The consultant prepared a report organizing and synthesizing the data and information, describing the analysis, and presenting written recommendations for action by staff and county health department leadership, plus local and state legislators. The comprehensive assessment data and research findings were used as evidence to convince the legislature to appropriate funding for the CHW program.

*Provision 8. The nurse collaborates with other health professionals and the public to protect human rights, promote health diplomacy, and reduce health disparities.*

ANA invited its members from across the nation to consider and address these questions:

- How should the nursing profession address incivility, bullying, and workplace violence in health care?
- Should nurses have the right to work in environments free from violence, environments that cut across the entire health care continuum and include both practice and academia?

Nurses, including PHNs, volunteered to serve on one of the largest committees to develop a position statement on incivility, bullying, and workplace violence. From a pool of more than 500 applicants, 4 co-chairs were chosen to lead a 24-member steering committee to develop the position statement. Collaborating with ANA staff members, the group also benefited from support from an advisory group of more than 400 nurse members representing various areas of nursing expertise, agencies, institutions, and regions of the country. *The ANA Position Statement on Incivility, Bullying and Workplace Violence* (ANA, 2015c) identifies the strong connection between what happens in the workplace and registered nurses'(RNs') health, patient safety, and nurse career consequences. The document is organized to include a review of the literature and historical background, definitions, a review of evidence, and the responsibilities of RNs and employers to create and support safe work environments. Recommended interventions across three levels of prevention are addressed in detail, including resources and potential strategies that might be operationalized in diverse agencies, institutions, organizations, and academic settings. A discussion of the relevant provisions of the ANA code of ethics is included, along with a lengthy list of references for further study (ANA, 2015c).

*Provision 9. The profession of nursing, collectively through its professional organizations, must articulate nursing values, maintain the integrity of the profession, and integrate principles of social justice into nursing and health policy.*

PHNs routinely serve on state and national organization and association legislative and policy committees that may propose legislation. With the support of the association's board of directors, the committees may seek legislative sponsors who can introduce bills intended to benefit the public's health, the nursing profession, or to advance nursing education. The committees also review proposed legislation and write memoranda in support of or opposition to the legislation.

Specialty and professional nurse association legislative and policy committees may take formal positions on proposed legislation. In some states, the relationship between the professional nurse association and legislators is strong, having grown to the point where legislators will first seek input and support from the committees prior to introducing legislation that might not garner nurse support. This relationship becomes essential, especially when attempts are made to pass legislation that might affect the state's nurse practice act, limit or expand the scope of nursing practice, or affect nursing education. Building a strong and positive relationship between the professional nurse association and legislators can effectively influence the development of all health policies, including those addressing public health issues, and ensure that social justice and equity are at the core.

## ADOPTING NEW AND EMERGING APPROACHES TO IMPROVE THE HEALTH OF POPULATIONS

PHNs have the necessary knowledge and experience to provide population-focused care that incorporates new and emerging approaches that can improve the health of populations.

### Genomics/Epigenetics

As scientists continue to seek to understand and explain the factors that prompt and affect the development of illness and manifestation of disease, 21st-century PHNs must become familiar with the specialized field of genetic epidemiology, known as *genomics*. Genomic risk factors contribute to development of illness and disease from a variety of environmental and occupational exposures.

*Epigenetics* is the study of how behaviors and environment can cause changes that affect the way one's genes work. Unlike genetic changes, epigenetic changes are reversible and do not change a person's DNA sequence, but they can change how a person's body reads a DNA sequence (CDC, 2020, August 3). Better understanding of genomic risk factors can help PHNs identify who is more likely to be affected by these exposures and guide targeted prevention efforts toward those most at risk. For example, there is a genetic role in several of the most prevalent noncommunicable diseases, including cancer, diabetes, cardiovascular disease, and asthma. Exploring the interplay among the environment, behavior, and genomic factors within and across populations will expand understanding of why some people experience illness and disease while others do not.

PHNs competent in their use of basic genomic information can help communities and policymakers understand the impact of genomics and family history on health outcomes. An emerging focus on precision medicine and precision public health holds promise for improvements in the ability not only to treat disease more effectively in individuals but to prevent disease and promote health in populations at risk. PHNs must use genomics with beneficence, without disenfranchising or limiting access to care for certain populations.

## Information Technology and Informatics

Historically, PHNs have always collected data about their populations' constituents. For example, Florence Nightingale is well known for her practice of gathering accurate morbidity and mortality data. From these raw data, she created colorful graphs that depicted the impact of sanitation and quality nursing care. Through data analysis, Nightingale translated the data into meaningful messages that would influence decision-making and development of care standards. Likewise, Lillian Wald, a well-known PH nursing pioneer, collected data through home visits and used it to compare data from several New York City hospitals. Her efforts were used to demonstrate that the care provided in the home setting improved client outcomes.

In today's health care environment, all PHNs must be competent in using information technology and informatics. At a minimum, PHNs need to demonstrate competence with use of the electronic health record (EHR), the personal health record (PHR), health information exchanges (HIE), and use of the Internet for secondary analysis of common population data sets and information, such as the census, morbidity and mortality data, and disease registries. Understanding such data and how to use relevant information systems improves the ability of PHNs to carry out the nursing process with the populations they serve.

For example, use of the electronic health record coupled with a geographic information system (GIS) can enhance the process that PHNs use during contact identification and tracking in a disease outbreak to determine where the cases may be clustered within a community. In this example, informatics brings data together, combines the data into a format that strengthens analysis, and graphically displays the data to increase meaning and understanding. The need to receive or share an individual's private health information to protect the health of the public creates a unique set of ethical issues for PHNs. It is important to note that although sharing of data for public health purposes has become much easier, there must be a specific focus on ensuring the privacy and security of this information.

### EVALUATION OF COMPETENCE

PHNs function within the domains of nursing, social, environmental, and public health sciences. Demonstration of competence associated with minimum standards in these areas is crucial to ensure that PH nursing practice is current, safe, grounded in evidence, and leads to the intended outcomes.

Multiple PHN-specific competency sets containing individual competencies that reflect demonstrated knowledge, skills, abilities, and judgment are available. Job-duty competency sets are specific to the knowledge and tasks required in a position or role. Core PHN competency sets are applicable across the specialty in any position or setting. Core PHN competency sets have distinguishing tiers or levels containing related practice-level competencies. Examples of core PHN competency sets include:

- *Essentials of Baccalaureate Nursing Education for Entry-Level Community/Public Health Nursing* (Association of Community Health Nursing Educators [ACHNE], 2010)
- *Entry-Level Population-Based Public Health Nursing Competencies* (Henry Street Consortium, 2017)
- *Community/Public Health Nursing Competencies* (QCC Competency Review Task Force, 2018): These competencies are divided into three tiers representing the direct service practice level, management or supervisory practice level, and senior or executive practice level, with strategic and systems-level responsibilities.
- This document, *Public Health Nursing: Scope and Standards of Practice, Third Edition,* delineates associated competencies for PH nursing practice and advanced PH nursing practice.

While it is ideal for PHNs to possess knowledge and skill in all competencies for their level or tier of practice, it is understood that certain positions may not expose PHNs to opportunities to achieve a high level of knowledge and skill for all competencies. PHNs should seek opportunities to develop knowledge and skills where they have identified gaps. In addition, competencies are cumulative in nature—i.e., demonstrated competence at higher levels or tiers occurs by building on accomplished lower-level competencies.

Evaluation of competence provides a baseline that reveals professional development needs and can be used to identify areas for individual performance improvement. Regular evaluation of competence allows PHNs to validate their current level of practice and provides a roadmap for addressing competency gaps and opportunities for growth. The timing of competence evaluation varies, depending on the PHN's employing organization, role, and experience. PHNs should receive formative and summative assessments and evaluations when learning new skills and critical behaviors and when orienting to new roles. At a minimum, an annual assessment or evaluation should occur to confirm the integrity and maintenance of requisite skills and critical behaviors. All assessments and evaluations should assess skills and critical behaviors in the three practice domains of nursing, social, and public health sciences.

The natural process of competence evaluation in PH nursing practice begins with self-assessment (Figure 4). This reflective practice is

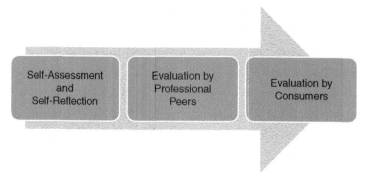

**Figure 4. Components of Competence Evaluation**

integral to the evaluative process and leads to the PHN's deeper understanding of the resulting practice appraisal. Evaluation by professional peers can be performed by a nurse peer, clinical instructor, supervisor, coach, mentor, or preceptor (ANA, 2015b). Consumers (individuals, families, groups, communities) should be invited to the evaluation process to share their unique perspective as recipients of PH nursing services.

Competence evaluation occurs in the practice setting through observation, return demonstration, and testing. What is evaluated depends on the PHN's role and level of practice. Characteristics of competence continually evolve as PH nursing practice progresses to address currently identified health care problems. Examples of foundational skills that should be regularly evaluated include clinical skills, translation of knowledge into practice (critical-thinking skills), strategic skills, and assessment and analytical skills. Examples of behaviors that can be evaluated include the use of tools and resources (quality improvement frameworks, evidence-based practice [EBP], current literature), community engagement, cultural competence, communication, and leadership.

No single standardized evaluation tool or process exists, as PH nursing roles vary by region and state. Although evaluation tools and processes can be built for specific settings, roles, and purposes (e.g., orientation, workforce development and training, performance evaluation), several reliable resources for competency assessment and validation are available through academic and professional sources. Table 1 summarizes four competency assessment resources commonly used in PH nursing practice.

Variability in PH nursing roles, settings, and competency evaluation tools and processes provides an opportunity for further exploration and development of effective competency evaluation methods. Having standardized evaluation methods that assess PH nursing competencies will lead to increased professional credibility and understanding of PH nursing practice.

**Table 1. Competency Evaluation Instruments**

| Tool | Source | Competency Focus |
|---|---|---|
| Competency Evaluation Tool (CET) | QCC for Public Health Nursing Organizations | Focus: PH nursing competencies in the domain of public health science<br><br>Developed as a template to assess *Tier 1 Community/Public Health Nursing Competencies*. Certification is also useful for evaluating PH nursing competencies and demonstrates that a minimum standard is met and maintained.<br><br>Level: May be adapted to fit individual skills, behaviors, tier or level of practice, and organizational needs specific to the PHN's role. (pp. 35–42) |
| Competencies for Public Health Nursing Practice Instrument (Version F) | University of Minnesota School of Nursing (Cross, S., Block, D., & Josten, L.) | Focus: Population-based PH nursing practice<br><br>This validity-tested instrument was developed to measure all aspects of population-based PH nursing practice. The instrument takes into consideration that skills change over time and that competence varies across practice areas.<br><br>Level: The tool is not structured to measure at a certain level or practice tier but to identify the skill level in each of the population-based practice areas of the instrument. |
| Competency Assessments for Public Health Professionals | Public Health Foundation: CoL Between Academia and Public Health Practice | Focus: Broad public health practice<br><br>Based on the 2014 version of the *Core Competencies for Public Health Professionals*, separate assessment tools are available for each of the three practice tiers, or levels, within the Core Competencies. The eight practice domains of the Core Competencies for Public Health Professionals are synonymous with the eight domains of the *Community/Public Health Nursing Competencies*.<br><br>Level: Competency assessments are available for three tiers or career stages for public health professionals (Tier 1, Frontline Staff/Entry Level; Tier 2, Program Management/Supervisory Level; Tier 3, Senior Management/Executive Level). |

**(Continued)**

**Table 1. Competency Evaluation Instruments (*Continued*)**

| Tool | Source | Competency Focus |
|---|---|---|
| Certification in Public Health (CPH) | National Board of Public Health Examiners | Focus: Foundational public health professional competencies |
| | | The Certification in Public Health is recognized as a valid public health professional credential. Baccalaureate-prepared PHNs with five years of public health experience are eligible to sit for the exam. Recertification requirements demonstrate commitment to the national standards through continuing education and professional development. |
| | | Level: Certification demonstrates that a public health professional has mastered 10 public health science domain areas that reflect essential practice competencies used in health department employment. |

# Public Health Nursing Practice Settings

PHNs provide care to people of all ages and health statuses. Their main focus is on assessing the health of populations and communities, ensuring access to care, promoting population health, and advocating for policy change domestically and internationally. Practice settings include but are not limited to clinics; local, state, and tribal government agencies; and health centers. PH nursing can be practiced anywhere there are human populations. Settings can be public health departments across cities, counties, states, and tribal nations; schools and universities; parishes and faith-based programs; home care; rural health; refugee and immigrant clinics; primary care clinics; jails and prisons; ambulatory outpatient facilities; voluntary organizations; hospitals; and a variety of community, public, and private agencies and organizations. Not all practice settings are defined by geographic or political boundaries when addressing the health of a population.

The practice environments for PHNs continue to evolve. PHNs with advanced education in research and/or practice can work within the academic setting, studying public health and PHN interventions and outcomes or educating the next generation of PHNs. Often, the work of PHNs overlaps with that of other health care professionals and community-based resources or in concert with multiple entities, providing system-level interventions in nontraditional settings (Carabez & Kim, 2019; Pittman, 2019).

The PHN's primary role is to promote, protect, and improve the health of the public. PHNs develop, supervise, manage, deliver, and evaluate services, programs, and initiatives focusing on the health of the population. They work in concert with multiple entities, such as hospitals, cities, counties, and states, in rural and urban settings to promote public health (Kub et al., 2017).

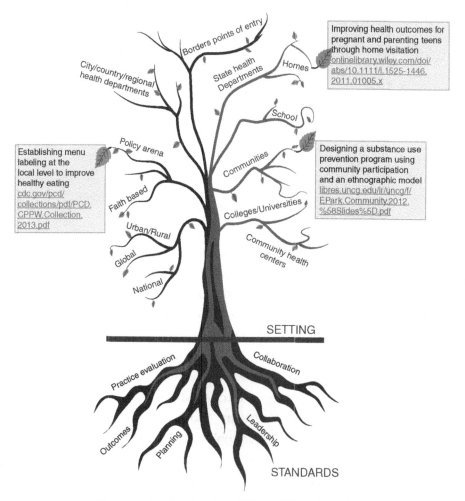

**Figure 5. Varied Settings Where PHNs Practice**

PHNs use a unique skill set to provide care in nontraditional settings as part of the *safety net*, the part of the health care system designed to protect vulnerable populations (LaHolt et al., 2018). Challenges to improving the health of the public are different in rural and frontier areas, where the PHN may be the only health care professional available for an entire county, with limited health care professional colleagues available for consultation (Bigbee et al., 2009).

In rural and urban settings, PHNs often have a broad scope of practice that includes communicable disease control/epidemiology and emergency preparedness. PHNs work to eliminate health inequities for those who have limited access to care, especially in rural areas (Abbott, 2014). PH nursing practice extends to schools and community programs (e.g., in advocacy for comprehensive sexual health education for adolescent populations; Dickson & Lobo, 2018).

In primary care, PHNs are members of the healthcare team who promote health and well-being (Josiah Macy Jr. Foundation, 2016). At the system level, PHNs are working interprofessionally within primary care clinics to promote health and well-being for patients and staff by translating health/disease guidelines, such as the Institute for Clinical Systems Improvement (ICSI) Adult Obesity Guideline and others, into practice (Monsen et al., 2015). PHNs can also work with hospitals to help meet their ACA 2010/IRS requirements for regular community health assessments (CHAs) or The Joint Commission accreditation standards for infectious disease prevention and control. Regardless of the setting, PHNs are valuable members or leaders of the health care team, working to promote, protect, and improve the health of the public.

# Characteristics of Public Health Nurses

## STATISTICAL SNAPSHOT

Nursing workforce data are collected in 35 states by established State Nursing Workforce Centers (National Forum of State Workforce Centers, 2019). Standardized minimum data sets are used by state boards of nursing related to the license renewal process to determine nursing supply and demand and educational preparation of nurses. Overall, these efforts and the associated data have provided some input on the composition and needs of the PH nursing workforce at a given time, but much more comprehensive regularly collected data are needed to better characterize PHNs. Systematic workforce data are not currently collected for PHNs.

In 2012, the Robert Wood Johnson Foundation contracted with the University of Michigan School of Public Health to conduct a survey of PHNs working in state and local health departments. Survey results revealed PHNs to be the largest occupational group of public health workers in these settings (Beck & Boulton, 2016). State and local health departments from 45 states employed approximately 34,521 full-time-equivalent RNs working in their settings. Educational background for the RNs was not consistently reported, but available data identified the diploma or associate's degree as the educational preparation for 31% of RNs; 51% had baccalaureate degrees in nursing; 10% had master's degrees or above; and the remaining 7% could not be identified from the data. The most common job classifications for nurses were PHN or community health nurse. RNs were also reported to be working in approximately 17 different program areas and 7 specific job function areas (see Appendix B for more details). Wide variation emerged in background experience, required education preparation, position titles, and salaries for RNs.

This study included additional surveys of a sample of individual RNs working in state and local health departments to determine job satisfaction, practice challenges and rewards, and respondent demographics. Of 7,500 RNs surveyed across all 50 states in state and local public health departments, 35% responded. More than 60% of the respondents were between the ages of 46 and 65 (Beck & Boulton, 2016). Major conclusions and recommendations from this survey included:

- The need to strengthen the education and training of PHNs;
- The provision of clinical services, which continues to be a major activity of RN in state and local health departments;
- The aging of the PHN workforce;
- Challenges in recruiting and hiring RNs into PH nursing positions;
- A lack of promotion opportunities for PHNs;
- A high level of job satisfaction among those employed as PHNs;
- A low level of satisfaction with salary; and
- The need for increasing the racial/ethnic diversity of PHNs to reflect the nation as a whole.

The University of Michigan Center for Excellence in Public Health Workforce Studies recommended that regular studies should be conducted to monitor the size, composition, capacity, and function of the PH nursing workforce through collaboration at the national, state, and practice levels. Such data should also include RNs functioning as PHNs but not working in governmental health agencies. In addition, projections of PHN staffing to meet state and local health needs could be useful for public health planning. Lastly, PHN job descriptions and performance reviews should be aligned with the *Public Health Nursing: Scope & Standards of Practice* and established PH nursing competencies (University of Michigan Center for Excellence in Public Health Workforce Studies, 2013).

## EDUCATION, CERTIFICATION, AND LICENSURE

Effective PH nursing practice requires PHNs to integrate knowledge from many disciplines in the delivery of nursing care with a population-based focus. The Quad Council (2018) recommends that the baccalaureate degree in nursing (Bachelor of Science in Nursing [BSN]) be the established educational preparation for entry-level PH nursing practice. BSN academic preparation includes an emphasis on health promotion and disease prevention at the population level, an essential component of improving population health (American Association of Colleges of Nursing [AACN], 2008). BSN programs are required to provide students with experiences in PH nursing. In addition, BSN-prepared nurses will have had required liberal arts coursework in the social sciences, enabling them to better identify and see the impact of SDOH. This educational background enables PHNs to demonstrate competence related to personal, social, policy, economic, work, and environmental determinants and how they affect the health status of individuals, communities, and populations (QCC Competency Review Task Force, 2018). Some states require a Bachelor of Science (BS) with a major in nursing for entry to practice as a PHN (New York: www.health.ny.gov/prevention/public_health_works/education/public_health_nurses.htm) or require additional education and certification (California: www.rn.ca.gov/pdfs/applicants/phn-app.pdf). However, there is currently no national legislative requirement for PHNs to have completed a BSN program.

The American Public Health Association, Public Health Nursing Section (2013), describes the role of the APHN as requiring the ability to synthesize public health and nursing science to promote the health of communities and populations. PHNs can become prepared for the practice at an advanced level through graduate education, including master's- or doctoral-level preparation in public health or PH nursing, in conjunction with on-the-job experience in roles of ever-increasing complexity and scope. Additional areas of educational focus may include public health ethics, public health administration, epidemiology, organizational theory, management theory, budget operations, grant/proposal writing, and program evaluation (Ervin & Kulbok, 2018). This preparation allows APHNs to hold leadership positions in governmental and nongovernmental organizations focused on public/population health. In such roles, APHNs develop population-level policies and interventions and ensure the implementation and evaluation of these initiatives.

Having a nursing clinical background and advanced public health/PH nursing education and experience has been documented to positively influence health outcomes of organizations (Bekemeier et al., 2012). Such a background prepares APHNs to serve in a leadership role when working with community groups, policymakers, and other components of the health care system on interventions to protect and maximize the health of the public, as envisioned in "Public Health 3.0: A Call to Action for Public Health to Meet the Challenges of the 21st Century" (DeSalvo et al., 2017).

PHNs in advanced practice, education, or research roles require graduate education and clinical practice related to PH nursing. Graduate education may be obtained through post-baccalaureate education in nursing or public health that now includes the Doctor of Nursing Practice (DNP) option, with specialization in community/public health nursing that focuses on community assessment, epidemiology, nursing theory, program planning, health advocacy, and policy. Other acceptable educational standards include (1) a Master's in Public Health (MPH) degree with a supervised nursing clinical practicum; (2) a graduate nursing degree with public health nursing specialty preparation; or

(3) a PH nursing certificate with courses in community assessment, nursing theory, nursing research, program planning, and a clinical practicum. A PHN educator or researcher with formal nursing education beyond the baccalaureate degree and a graduate public health degree integrates principles from nursing and public health for teaching excellence and advancing the science of PH nursing (Dupin et al., 2020; Shaw et al., 2016). Additional areas of educational focus may include ethics for PH nursing. It is also important that clinicians and educators have clinical experience in health promotion/disease prevention, community assessment, program planning/management, and evaluation at the population level.

According to the AACN, 13 universities offered a DNP in advanced public health nursing in 2019, with an average enrollment of 11 students. Four DNP programs were identified in population health nursing, with an average enrollment of 18 students. At the master's level, 34 universities offered programs in community/public health nursing, with an average enrollment of 33 students in 2019; however, this number was skewed by one school that recorded an enrollment of more than 357 students, while an additional six schools recorded enrollments of fewer than 5 students (AACN, 2020).

Certification in PH nursing is not currently available at the PHN or APHN practice level. However, PHNs can be certified in public health through the National Board of Public Health Examiners (National Board of Public Health Examiners [NBPHE], n.d.). For APHNs, certification by the American Nurses Credentialing Center (ANCC) was terminated in 2017 due to small numbers of applicants. However, those previously certified by ANCC as APHNs (PHNA-BC, PHCNS-BC) may continue to renew their certifications every five years through the ANCC. Because PHNs have such a wide scope of practice across individual, community, and systems levels, other existing certifications can serve to document discrete knowledge and skills relevant to PH nursing practice, but none of these certifications addresses the full scope of PHN or APHN practice. (See Appendix C for other relevant certifications for PHNs.)

All PHNs are required to hold an active, unencumbered nursing license.

# Current Trends and Challenges for Public Health Nursing

PH nursing practice in the US is dynamic and becoming increasingly complex. Societal and political changes in the 21st century have enhanced this evolution. Identified threats to the health of populations include but are not limited to:

- The re-emergence of communicable diseases and increasing incidence of drug-resistant organisms;
- Environmental hazards, including air and water pollution and climate change;
- Physical or civic barriers to healthy lifestyles (e.g., food "deserts");
- Overall concern about the structure and function of the health care system;
- Modern public health epidemics, such as obesity, pandemic influenza and SARS, COVID-19, tobacco-related diseases and deaths, violence, and the substance-use disorders and opioid crises;
- Global and emerging crises, with increased opportunities for exposure to multiple health threats;
- Decreases in US life expectancy; and
- Systemic racism and structural injustice.

These and other threats have highlighted a dramatic need for enhancing the nation's public health all-hazards preparedness, with the goal of enhancing response and recovery. PHNs have knowledge and skills in activities centered on preparedness, such as community-wide syndromic surveillance, triage, and coordination of disaster health services and shelters; the handling of biological and chemical agents; as well as the removal or reduction of public health hazards. PHNs use this skill set in innovative partnerships with community-level organizations and groups to prepare and protect people, communities, and populations.

As priority public health initiatives evolve to address emerging health trends, PHNs often assume leadership roles as needed. They identify evidence to support public health systems' changes and implement and evaluate those changes. PH nursing leadership ultimately enhances the ability of public health systems to address the health and social issues facing all people and creates conditions in which people can be healthy (Bekemeier et al., 2012).

PH nursing practice changes and evolves with new health challenges, changes in the health care system, and current technological, social, and environmental trends. Such changes include but are not limited to continually evolving technology needs, nurse entrepreneurship opportunities, interprofessional collaboration partnerships, health care financing (e.g., Medicaid transformation/expansion changes, Patient Protection and Affordable Care Act, value-based payments, available grant funding, etc.), and replacing PHNs with less expensive non-nursing staff in key areas.

## SOCIETAL CHANGES

The loss of a sense of community has emerged as the US has moved from the industrial era to the information age (LaChance, 2014; Quinones, personal communication, May 10, 2019). PHNs can address this growing trend and partner with others to restore personal and community responsibility (Florez, 2007). For example, new data from WHO suggest that 23 million of the world's children did not receive recommended vaccines during 2020 (WHO, 2021). The anti-vaccination movement is not a new trend: people have been objecting to vaccinations since their inception. Despite comprehensive scientific evidence to support vaccination, the anti-vaccination movement continues to grow. In part, that growth can be attributed to social media as a platform for rapid, expansive distribution of incorrect information and vaccination myths. PHNs are challenged to respond with appropriate, effective communications and dissemination of enhanced educational information.

Globalization and mass migration hold huge implications for global health (Gostin & Friedman, 2017). Global travel and immigration provide vehicles for pandemic outbreaks of life-threatening disease, such as the Ebola virus (Cohen et al., 2016), COVID-19, and difficult to treat microbes, such as drug-resistant tuberculosis (MacPherson et al., 2007). In many countries, the existing infrastructure for caring for their populace is often insufficient to address these global health issues, and a more integrated, international approach is warranted (MacPherson et al., 2007). PHNs are essential in establishing a global network of public health professionals ready to collaborate and share warnings, resources, and solutions.

## Systemic Racism

PHNs recognize the pernicious effect of systemic racism on health equity. Current systemic inequities, structural barriers, and health disparities—individually, institutionally, and structurally—reflect the long-standing historical and pervasive impact of systemic racism on SDOH and the health of marginalized populations. Health policies can design solutions to address health outcomes, health care financing, and health care delivery (Castle et al., 2019; Keys, 2021; Kett, 2020). PHNs can leverage their knowledge of working with communities or specific population groups and participation in assessing and evaluating health services to address structural competency, structural injustice, and systemic racism. Through interprofessional collaborative practice, PHNs are uniquely poised to help overcome systemic racism and structural injustice. With the ever-complex health care system and long-standing racial hierarchy, the need will continue for PHNs to assist with collaboratively working at the systems and policy levels, community level, and interpersonal level to address systemic racism and to facilitate processes to advance health equity (Broussard et al., 2020).

## Regulatory Authority and Public Health Emergencies

It is vital to have an adequate public health infrastructure in place, with a well-educated public health workforce that is prepared to monitor and protect the public's health as the need arises (Baker & Koplan, 2002). For example, the Environmental Protection Agency (EPA) is a regulatory entity with the legal authority to enforce regulations addressing a variety of human and environmental health concerns (US Environmental Protection Agency [USEPA], 2016). The US Congress enacted the Safe Drinking Water Act in 1974. Under this act, "the EPA retains national oversight responsibility for state administration and enforcement" and has "emergency authority to address imminent and substantial endangerment to human health from drinking water contamination" (USEPA, 2016, p. 2). In 1994, the EPA administrator delegated the authority to issue emergency orders to regional administrators. Publicly available data indicate that most emergency orders have been issued "to businesses and federal facilities" (USEPA, 2016, p. 6). These emergency orders are not always sufficient to protect the health of the public. Environmental health and advocacy present growing challenges for PH nursing practice and for safeguarding the public's health.

## Political Determinants of Health

The SARS-CoV2 pandemic has exacerbated the health inequities that already existed in the US. Dawes has identified that "racial and ethnic minorities are disproportionately impacted by the global pandemic" (2020, p. 78) and are far more likely to die from COVID-19 than are other populations.

According to Dawes (2020), political determinants of health often underlie health inequities. The political determinants of health create social drivers that affect health and create structural barriers to equity for particular populations lacking power and privilege. Thus, health inequities are created when a system has not valued each group equally and when social services, health care services, and other opportunities have been distributed inequitably. This failure to value everyone equally has left certain groups with lower health status, which becomes even more magnified during crises, such as a pandemic.

Dawes (2020) claims that to achieve equity in all health policies, we must first harness the political process that creates policies and implement policies that value equity (as fairness) and social justice. Furthermore, Dawes states that to elevate health equity in this way, the political determinants of health—the very policies that underlie and create inequities in the first place—must be addressed.

Dawes (2018) describes previous examples of policies in US history intended to address health disparities and inequities. These examples include Medicaid and Medicare, which continue to survive today. However, the ACA (2010) is the longest-surviving health reform law in America to specifically prioritize health equity. Its intent was to create a more accessible, equitable, and inclusive health system. Its very survival depends on harnessing future political processes and policies.

## Education for Public Health Nursing Roles

The PH nursing specialty experiences a significant challenge in adequately preparing nurses for practice at both PHN and APHN levels. This challenge is due, in part, to the reality that a substantial proportion of the PH nursing workforce nationwide does not possess a minimum preparation of a baccalaureate degree. In addition, many PHNs practicing at an advanced level in community organizations and health departments do not possess a minimum of a master's degree or any graduate-level education in public health/public health nursing (APHA, 2013).

The QCC (2018) developed a set of PHN practice competencies that are leveled and specify the roles and responsibilities associated with each of three tiers. Although this competency set helps with educating and evaluating PH nursing practice, it is not used extensively. Little et al. (2019) have surveyed a convenience sample of PHNs in practice and education, with results indicating that 40% of the respondents were unaware of or did not use the QCC competencies. In addition, there is no external certification or recognition of PH nursing knowledge and skills, unlike many other nursing specialties that have such external certifications or recognitions.

## Evolving Nursing Education Models

Nursing education models are constantly evolving as new technologies are developed, and virtual nursing education platforms continue to expand. One thing that will not change is the need for highly educated nurses to respond to 21st-century health challenges (IOM, 2011). Desired 21st-century nursing competencies identified in IOM's *Future of Nursing* report (2011) address leadership, health policy, quality improvement, research and evidence-based practice, teamwork and collaboration, and specific content areas, such as community and public health. These competencies must also include ethics, technology skills, and familiarity with information management systems.

The widely accepted entry level for nursing practice, and particularly PH nursing practice, is the BS, with a major in nursing. The rapidly growing numbers of online nursing education programs offering RN-BS bridge programs play a key role in helping advance nursing education to the level required for entry into PH nursing practice. Research shows that nursing education programs are adopting new technology at a faster pace than general education (Siwicki, 2017). Both nurses and employers benefit. Virtual classrooms with asynchronous educational activities allow nurses to continue full-time employment in nursing while also pursuing an advanced level of education. From the employer perspective, virtual nursing education programs help keep the current nursing workforce in active practice, while nurses concurrently increase their education and skills for delivering higher quality care (Siwicki, 2017). These nursing programs must continue to include core PH nursing content.

Increasing the number of nurses with BSNs also opens the door for further education for graduate and doctoral degrees, allowing nurses to serve as APHNs, primary care providers, nurse researchers, and nurse faculty (IOM, 2011). Additional resources and learning opportunities must be committed to ensure that nurses are life-long learners with multiple venues for continuing education activities and advanced certifications for specific practice areas. Nurse residency programs are valuable mechanisms for providing requisite hands-on experience for transitions in practice.

The 2011 *Future of Nursing* report was successful in facilitating many nursing accomplishments during the last decade, including increasing the number of baccalaureate-prepared nurses, decreasing practice barriers, and accelerating the role of nurses in leadership positions (Stringer, 2019). Those changes were largely internal to the nursing profession and its practice and workforce preparation. Further work is required to assess and enhance nursing's contribution to the health of the public.

## *Future of Nursing 2020–2030*

The delayed *Future of Nursing 2020–2030* study has been completed and published (National Academies of Science, Engineering, and Medicine [NASEM], 2021). The Robert Wood Johnson Foundation again partnered with NASEM to extend the vision for the nursing profession into 2030 and chart a path for the nursing profession to help the US create a culture of health, reduce health disparities, and improve the health and well-being of its population in the 21st century. This edition of the *Future of*

*Nursing* focused externally on nursing's contributions to the health of the public, particularly nursing roles in assessing and addressing SDOH. PHNs are well positioned to lead this endeavor.

## Population Health Management

The National Advisory Council on Nursing Education and Practice published *Preparing Nurses for Roles in Population Health Management* in 2016. This report emphasizes the foundational knowledge about population health management that PHNs and APHNs hold and integrate into practice. Population health, including population health management, is gaining importance as a pillar in nursing education and practice. Recent work funded by the Robert Wood Johnson Foundation has examined nursing education and practice in population health (Gorski et al., 2019).

## Healthy People 2030

*The Healthy People 2030* framework for action that builds on the *Healthy People 2020* platform can serve as a guide for nursing practice. The Healthy People initiative is a federal program that provides "science-based, 10-year national objectives for improving the health of all Americans." For the past 40 years, Healthy People has monitored the health of Americans and set benchmarks for how all can be healthier. Guided by health promotion and disease prevention criteria, with measurable objectives and goals, states and localities are invited to use the national framework and objectives to develop their own plans.

Although its focus has always been health promotion and disease prevention, the *Healthy People 2020* agenda was the first to use SDOH to frame the conceptual understanding of health, health promotion, and disease prevention. These underpinnings are the essence that guides programming often developed and executed by the PH nursing workforce. In support of *Healthy People 2030*, the interprofessional Association for Prevention Teaching and Research Healthy People Curriculum Task Force has updated *The Clinical Prevention and Population Health Curriculum Framework*, a valuable resource for PHNs in practice and faculty teaching clinical prevention and population health (Association for Prevention Teaching and Research [APTR], 2020).

Additionally, *The Community Guide* developed by the federal Community Preventive Services Task Force "is a collection of evidence-based findings...[of] interventions to improve health and prevent disease" for use by states, communities, organizations, businesses, health care organizations, or schools (Community Preventive Services Task Force [CPSTF], 2020). PHNs use this resource to help select evidence-based interventions for programs and services that address population health.

## TITLE VIII FUNDING

The PH nursing specialty area provides a foundation for planning and evaluating community/public health programs. Content includes learning about community/public health concepts, health promotion, population-level interventions, grant writing, health care systems, leadership, and health policy; addressing health inequities of vulnerable and diverse populations; and practicing and consulting in diverse and multicultural settings. The Health Resources and Services Administration (HRSA) offers a number of funding opportunities for the development of programs centered on improving the health of specific populations while enhancing the nursing workforce and leadership. These include the Nurse Education, Practice, Quality, and Retention (NEPQR) Program; the Advanced Nursing Education Workforce (ANEW) program; and the Nursing Workforce Diversity (NWD) program. APHNs have served as developers, project directors, and in other leadership roles in these innovative programs. However, funding in the past decade for the Advanced Nursing Education program has been limited to nurse practitioner programs, thus eliminating this support for nurses seeking advanced education in PH nursing.

PH nursing is well positioned to play an important part in the Robert Wood Johnson Foundation's Culture of Health strategies to lead nursing toward creating a culture of health, reducing health disparities, and improving population health in the 21st century (Robert Wood Johnson Foundation [RWJF], 2019, 2021).

Although it is difficult to fully predict the direction of nursing in the coming decade and beyond, there are currently many issues for PHNs to consider, including, but not limited to:

- Addressing the social and environmental determinants of health and documenting results;
- Ensuring the provision of high-quality, affordable health care;
- Promoting social and environmental justice;
- Researching the comparative effectiveness of health care delivery models;
- Enhancing nursing workforce diversity, equity, and inclusion;
- Promoting APHN education;
- Measuring the impact of PH nursing and advanced PH nursing practice;
- Enhancing nursing's health and well-being (i.e., taking care of our own);
- Advancing the appropriate use of technology to promote health;
- Improving pandemic and emergency preparedness; and
- Advancing health equity in all policies and practice.

## Summary of Scope of Public Health Nursing Practice

As the health care system moves toward acknowledging and addressing the multiple factors that influence health, public health becomes an ever-more-critical partner, having long promoted this view of health within the context of communities and in all policies. PHNs are uniquely positioned to lead these efforts as the nursing specialty that bridges the clinical role of nursing and the broader community role of public health. PHNs can educate other nurses in basic population health knowledge and skills for care across the health care continuum. Additionally, PHNs practice at the community and population levels and across sectors, focusing on enhancing health equity by improving access to care, social and environmental conditions, and health policies. To do this, however, PHNs need to clearly identify and embrace their specialty and its standards and demonstrate the competencies needed to practice effectively. The next section outlines specific practice standards and accompanying competencies at the PHN and APHN levels of practice.

# Standards of Public Health Nursing Practice

The Standards of Public Health Nursing Practice are authoritative statements of the actions and behaviors that all public health nurses (PHN), regardless of role, population, and setting, are expected to perform competently. These published standards may serve as evidence of the standard of practice, with the understanding that the application of the standards and accompanying competencies depends on context, circumstances, or situation.

The standards are subject to change with the dynamics of the nursing profession as evidence is discovered and new patterns of professional practice are developed and accepted by the nursing profession and the public. In addition, specific conditions and clinical circumstances may affect the application of the standards at a given time (e.g., during a natural disaster, epidemic, or pandemic). The standards are subject to formal, periodic review and revision.

## Significance of Standards

The Standards of Public Health Nursing Practice describe a competent level of nursing practice as organized by the critical-thinking model known as the *nursing process*. The nursing process includes the components of assessment, diagnosis, outcomes identification, planning, implementation, and evaluation. Accordingly, the nursing process encompasses significant actions taken by PHNs and forms the foundation of the nurse's decision-making, practice, and provision of care.

The Standards of Professional Performance describe a competent level of behavior in the professional role, including activities related to ethics; respectful and equitable practice; communication; collaboration; leadership; education; evidence-based practice (EBP) and research; quality of practice; professional practice appraisal; resource utilization; environmental health, planetary health, and environmental justice; and advocacy. All PHNs are expected to engage in professional activities, including leadership, reflective of their education, position, and role. PHNs are accountable for their professional actions to themselves, health care consumers, peers, and, ultimately, society.

## The Function of Competencies in Standards

A *competency* is an expected level of performance that integrates knowledge, skills, abilities, and judgment (ANA, 2014). The competencies that accompany each standard are applicable to all licensed PHNs. The numbering sequence is used for identification and does not reflect a hierarchy or prioritization. Where appropriate, additional discrete competencies applicable to advanced public health nurses (APHNs) are identified with the addition of *A* following the assigned number. The competencies that accompany each standard may be evidence of demonstrated compliance with the corresponding standard. The list of competencies is not exhaustive.

A registered nurse entering the public health nursing (PH nursing) specialty, whether as a new graduate or after working in a non-PH nursing setting, will need further experience and education (academic or continuing professional development) to achieve and demonstrate competence in PH nursing.

PHNs work with individuals, families, and groups—always within the context of a population/community. PHNs may have additional opportunities or assignments that include working directly with communities or populations, although that may not be common for all PHNs.

APHNs at a minimum work with communities and populations and hold advanced degrees and certifications, and/or extensive years of public health experience and professional development. APHNs are expected to demonstrate competence as reflected in both the PHN-level competencies and additional advanced-level competencies.

**IMPORTANT:** Recognition, licensure, and scope of practice of the registered nurse vary by state, commonwealth, and territory. Therefore, PHNs must always be familiar with their jurisdiction's nurse practice act, laws, and regulations governing nursing practice.

# Standards of Practice

## STANDARD 1. ASSESSMENT

The PHN collects comprehensive data pertinent to the health status of populations.

### Competencies

The PHN:

**1.1.** Describes systematic and comprehensive population-focused assessment as a primary focus of PHN practice.

**1.2.** Recognizes that population-focused assessments can vary in scope (e.g., community, population-specific, neighborhood-specific, etc.) and focus (e.g., comprehensive, assets, needs, etc.).

**1.3.** Assesses the social determinants of health (SDOH), including assets; needs; values; beliefs; resources; and relevant social, political, and environmental factors.

**1.4.** Assesses health status, health literacy, disparities and inequities, and public health conditions.

**1.5.** Uses assessment data and priorities as bases for planning, developing, implementing, and evaluating interventions to address identified health issues.

**1.6.** Participates in planning a community assessment using principles of community engagement (CE), PH nursing, social ecology, and a systems perspective.

**1.7.** Identifies potential partners, at-risk populations, stakeholders, and community members when developing the partnership to guide the assessment process.

**1.8.** Identifies variables that reflect an ecological perspective to measure SDOH, health status, and public health conditions of the populations, communities, groups, families, or individuals.

**1.9.** Uses a data collection plan that incorporates valid and reliable methods and instruments from nursing, public health, natural, social, and applied sciences for collecting qualitative and quantitative data from appropriate sources.

**1.10.** Addresses barriers and limitations to comprehensive data collection.

**1.11.** Analyzes assessment data using evidence-based models and techniques from nursing, epidemiology, biostatistics, demography, and other sciences.

**1.12.** Synthesizes data analysis results to enable interpretation of findings and formulation of conclusions about health status, health outcomes, inequities, and public health conditions.

**1.13.** Demonstrates compliance with privacy, confidentiality, ethical, legal, and policy standards, principles, and guidelines of PH nursing, public health, and other regulatory bodies in matters related to assessment data and information collection.

## Additional Competencies for the Advanced Public Health Nurse

In addition to the competencies for the PHN, the APHN:

**1.14A.** Partners with community members, health professionals, and other stakeholders to identify a comprehensive set of relevant variables within and across systems to measure determinants of health, health status, and public health conditions.

**1.15A.** Adopts a comprehensive set of relevant variables within and across systems to measure health and public health conditions.

**1.16A.** Addresses gaps, redundancies, and other limitations in assessment data.

**1.17A.** Maximizes information technology resources in collaboration with others in the design of assessment data collection processes.

**1.18A.** Engages with community members, partners, health professionals, and other stakeholders to attach shared meaning to collected data.

**1.19A.** Analyzes qualitative and quantitative assessment data in partnership with community members, partners, health professionals, and other stakeholders using evidence-based principles and models from nursing, public health, social, natural, and applied sciences.

**1.20A.** Synthesizes qualitative and quantitative assessment data in partnership with community members, partners, health professionals, and other stakeholders using evidence-based principles and models from nursing, public health, social, natural, and applied sciences.

**1.21A.** Partners with community members, health professionals, and other stakeholders to prioritize assessment findings to support the development of population diagnoses and population-focused plans.

**1.22A.** Collaborates with the community and other public health professionals, partners, health professionals, stakeholders, and the interdisciplinary team to evaluate the design, management, and sharing of public health system data that focus on population health status, assets, needs, and concerns.

# STANDARD 2. DIAGNOSIS

The PHN analyzes assessment data to determine actual or potential diagnoses, problems, and issues related to health and well-being.

## Competencies

The PHN:

**2.1.** Develops PH nursing diagnoses to guide planning of interventions to address risks or needs prioritized from analysis and interpretation of assessment data.

**2.2.** Uses an ecological perspective and epidemiological data to identify health and safety risks and barriers.

**2.3.** Incorporates assessment data from a variety of sources to formulate diagnoses, problems, and issues.

**2.4.** Uses varied approaches to identify community needs and strengths to integrate community preferences into the diagnoses.

**2.5.** Prioritizes diagnoses, problems, and issues based on mutually established goals to meet health care consumer needs.

**2.6.** Demonstrates a variety of documentation methods to disseminate diagnoses, problems, issues, and public health information.

## Additional Competencies for the Advanced Public Health Nurse

In addition to the competencies of the PHN, the APHN:

**2.7A.** Develops diagnoses to guide planning of systems level interventions to address risks or needs prioritized from analysis and interpretation of assessment data.

**2.8A.** Determines diagnoses that affect program planning and evaluation, staff development, interprofessional teamwork, and other organizational activities.

# STANDARD 3. OUTCOMES IDENTIFICATION

The PHN identifies expected outcomes for a plan specific to the health status of the population or the situation.

## Competencies

The PHN:

**3.1.** Involves individuals, families, organizations, stakeholders, and members of the interprofessional health care team in formulating expected outcomes.

**3.2.** Uses formal and informal networks among health care professionals, community organizations, and health systems in formulating expected outcomes.

**3.3.** Involves key stakeholders and resources necessary in identifying expected outcomes for collective impact on improving the health of diverse and underserved populations.

**3.4.** Considers evidence from practice and research in identifying expected outcomes.

**3.5.** Identifies the expected outcomes that reflect shared values through CE that are understandable to all involved entities.

**3.6.** Identifies SDOH in formulating appropriate outcomes across the lifespan.

**3.7.** Identifies local, state, national, and international policies relevant to the health of individuals, families, and communities in determining acceptable, accessible, and achievable expected outcomes for all.

**3.8.** Develops expected outcomes that reflect a long-term commitment to enhancing population health.

**3.9.** Participates in quality-improvement processes within an established timeline for achieving expected outcomes for individuals, families, groups, and communities.

## Additional Competencies for the Advanced Public Health Nurse

In addition to the competencies for the PHN, the APHN:

**3.10A.** Develops an established timeline for achieving expected outcomes.

**3.11A.** Uses technology effectively to collect, store, analyze, and retrieve data related to expected outcomes.

**3.12A.** Incorporates EBP and knowledge of available resources; environmental factors; ethical, legal, and privacy considerations; and time estimates in defining expected outcomes.

**3.13A.** Identifies relevant health policy that addresses expected outcomes.

**3.14A.** Defines evidence-based expected outcomes that are efficient, effective, and aligned with practice and community partners.

**3.15A.** Incorporates evidence-based strategies to identify expected outcomes that modify systems of care.

**3.16A.** Incorporates system-level interventions, satisfaction of stakeholders, the population, the organization, and the resolution of health concerns in identifying expected outcomes.

**3.17A.** Develops expected outcomes for programmatic budget priorities based on stakeholder needs, cost analysis, and financial input from federal, state, tribal, and local sources.

**3.18A.** Develops organization-wide budgets to provide resources to meet the needs of individuals, families, and communities when defining expected outcomes.

**3.19A.** Uses organizational strategic plans and other resources in determining expected outcomes.

**3.20A.** Uses formal and informal networks among health care professionals, community organizations, and health systems in evaluating expected outcomes.

# STANDARD 4. PLANNING

The PHN develops plans that prescribe strategies to attain optimal health and well-being.

## Competencies

The PHN:

**4.1.** Uses assessment findings to support planning that reflects the definition of health as a shared value.

**4.2.** Uses assessments to plan and develop evidence-based community programs.

**4.3.** Partners with community members, health professionals, and other stakeholders to prioritize assessment findings, diagnoses or problems, and outcomes to support the development of population-focused plans.

**4.4.** Demonstrates prioritization of "level of risk" based on SDOH to advance health.

**4.5.** Uses evidenced-based strategies and tools, including data, to plan for (1) health promotion and restoration; (2) prevention of illness, disease, and injury; (3) alleviation of suffering; and (4) supportive care.

**4.6.** Contributes to program planning that reflects evidence-based strategies in identifying expected outcomes.

**4.7.** Incorporates evidence-based guidelines and pathways to operationalize the PH nursing process.

**4.8.** Demonstrates budget and cost implication knowledge according to economic trends while engaging in program planning.

**4.9.** Develops program plans that are compliant with laws, statutes, regulations, and standards of care relevant to PH nursing practice.

**4.10.** Recognizes the need for program plan refinement according to a quality-improvement framework based on outcomes.

**4.11.** Uses standard language, recognized terminology, and/or plain language to document program plan outcomes and disseminate results to stakeholders and communities of interest.

**4.12.** Advocates for nursing care and CE that are reflective of culture, values, and ethical concerns.

**4.13.** Modifies the plan based on appropriate health behavior change theory, new knowledge, population response, or other relevant factors to achieve expected outcomes.

## Additional Competencies for the Advanced Public Health Nurse

In addition to the competencies of the PHN, the APHN:

**4.14A.** Uses evidence-based tools and epidemiologic data to develop methodologic program plans that also address evaluation.

**4.15A.** Uses epidemiological data, concepts, and other evidence to analyze SDOH when developing and tailoring population-level health services.

**4.16A.** Uses system-level methods, planning models, epidemiology, and other analytic processes to develop, implement, and evaluate population-level interventions that address (1) health promotion; (2) prevention of illness, injury, or disease; (3) suffering; and (4) emergency preparedness and response.

**4.17A.** Includes models, theories, policy, and best available evidence to address specific public health issues across the lifespan.

**4.18A.** Creates meaningful opportunities for collaborative programming among community partners, focusing on shared vision, values, and principles for community action.

**4.19A.** Develops partnerships with members of the interprofessional team, stakeholders, and communities of interest when planning health care policies, programs, and services.

**4.20A.** Applies current policy, regulation, standards, and statutes to the planning process.

**4.21A.** Modifies program plans through ongoing assessment of population outcomes.

**4.22A.** Uses SDOH data and information to guide program planning that is culturally sensitive and understandable for the communities of interest.

**4.23A.** Uses program-planning skills and community-based participatory research (CBPR; i.e., collaboration, reflection, capacity building) to engage marginalized/disadvantaged populations in making decisions that affect their health and well-being.

# STANDARD 5. IMPLEMENTATION

The PHN implements identified plans.

## Competencies
The PHN:

**5.1.** Engages individuals, families, communities, and population resources in implementing interprofessional collaborative programs that address the assessed/identified health needs present within a community.

**5.2.** Delivers PH nursing evidence-based services to promote health.

**5.3.** Enables systems and resources during the implementation of culturally appropriate services.

**5.4.** Delivers evidence-based, culturally responsive services.

**5.5.** Integrates the ecological perspective when implementing plans with diverse individuals, families, communities, and populations.

**5.6.** Integrates conceptual frameworks for action on SDOH in implementing programs.

**5.7.** Uses appropriate technology to collect, analyze, store, and retrieve data as evidence prior to implementing or promoting EBP.

## Additional Competencies for the Advanced Public Health Nurse

In addition to the competencies for the PHN, the APHN:

**5.8A.** Develops tailored population-level health services based on concise, comprehensive community/population assessments and the collection, analysis, and interpretation of qualitative, quantitative, epidemiological, and archival data in conjunction with surveillance data.

**5.9A.** Incorporates formative evaluation during implementation of the plan.

# STANDARD 5A. COORDINATION OF CARE

The PHN coordinates care delivery.

## Competencies

The PHN:

**5A.1.** Promotes coordinated policies, programs, and services for goal attainment relevant to population health.

**5A.2.** Incorporates care management that includes broad community coordination of public health services.

**5A.3.** Conducts surveillance, outreach, screening, case finding, and other functions with diverse stakeholders to enhance delivery of public health services.

**5A.4.** Connects individuals, groups, and populations with needed public health care and services.

**5A.5.** Follows up on referrals for public health services, interventions, and care delivery.

**5A.6.** Documents activities and actions taken to support access to care and coordination of care and services.

**5A.7.** Applies best practices to ensure effective PH nursing care delivery.

**5A.8.** Identifies local, state, national, and global policy issues relevant to coordinating public health services to improve well-being.

**5A.9.** Provides information to inform policy decisions related to the equitable distribution and delivery of public health services and care.

**5A.10.** Gathers input from stakeholders when delivering coordinated public health care services.

**5A.11.** Collects data and evidence that incorporate qualitative, quantitative, and experiential data, along with narrative evidence, to inform and improve public health service delivery and care coordination.

**5A.12.** Bases coordinated health care service delivery approaches on identified community and population needs, strengths, and capacities that can be tailored to achieve equity.

**5A.13.** Applies a variety of methods to disseminate timely and trustworthy public health information regarding available public health services and care coordination.

## Additional Competencies for the Advanced Public Health Nurse

In addition to the competencies for the PHN, the APHN:

**5A.14A.** Provides leadership and oversight for the coordination of health care service delivery within and across systems, agencies, organizations, and jurisdictions.

**5A.15A.** Synthesizes information, data, and evidence to prescribe the necessary systems and community support measures to meet desired goals.

**5A.16A.** Addresses ongoing and emerging issues related to critical life stages.

**5A.17A.** Prioritizes empirical evidence indicating insufficient well-being at critical points across the lifespan in specific populations to equitably distribute limited benefits and resources.

**5A.18A.** Applies diverse theoretical perspectives to guide the coordination of system-wide approaches to reduce population and community health risks and improve health and well-being.

**5A.19A.** Maximizes effective communication regarding integrated care delivery with systems leaders, community anchors, and key stakeholders.

**5A.20A.** Designs systems to support quantitative, qualitative, and experiential data and evidence to ensure coordinated health care service delivery and promotion of population well-being.

**5A.21A.** Evaluates system-wide health care delivery guidelines, processes, and structures to promote equity and structural justice.

# STANDARD 5B. HEALTH TEACHING AND HEALTH PROMOTION

The PHN employs multiple strategies to promote health and safety.

## Competencies
The PHN:

**5B.1.** Uses available data and resources related to SDOH when conducting health education, health promotion, risk reduction, and disease prevention programs and services for individuals, families, and groups.

**5B.2.** Incorporates input from individuals, families, and groups when planning and delivering health care programs and services.

**5B.3.** Incorporates research evidence or promising practices to promote health in communities and populations.

**5B.4.** Selects teaching and learning methods using appropriate health literacy strategies and focused on the population's identified needs, objectives, and resources.

**5B.5.** Provides anticipatory guidance with information about intended effects and potential adverse effects of proposed programs and services.

**5B.6.** Uses data, evidence, and information technology to understand the impact of determinants of health.

## Additional Competencies for the Advanced Public Health Nurse

In addition to the competencies for the PHN, the APHN:

**5B.7A.** Implements population-level health teaching and health promotion interventions.

**5B.8A.** Designs health promotion and disease prevention educational programs based on the literacy level of the population served.

**5B.9A.** Modifies existing health education and health promotion programs based on feedback from participants, providers, health professionals, and other stakeholders.

**5B.10A.** Uses empirical evidence and relevant theories and frameworks when designing health teaching and health promotion programs.

**5B.11A.** Engages relevant stakeholders in health teaching and health promotion activities.

**5B.12A.** Leads nurses and other health professionals in planning and coordinating evidence-based health teaching and health promotion programs and services.

# STANDARD 5C. CONSULTATION

The PHN provides consultation to enhance the abilities of diverse stakeholders to create and effect change.

## Competencies

The PHN:

**5C.1.** Consults within and across systems and with individuals, families, groups, populations, and communities.

**5C.2.** Seeks local community knowledge and community member and leader involvement in identifying needs, generating solutions, setting priorities, planning to address public health and social issues, and evaluating outcomes.

**5C.3.** Demonstrates understanding of groups, group dynamics, and group development.

**5C.4.** Actively and openly seeks to learn from and with stakeholders.

**5C.5.** Creates spaces and opportunities for stakeholder growth and active participation.

**5C.6.** Operates from a position of belief and trust in participating stakeholders.

**5C.7.** Actively attends to stakeholder contributions, questions, and concerns.

**5C.8.** Provides testimony and professional opinion on public health issues, programs, policies, and services.

**5C.9.** Communicates consultation recommendations and evidence to relevant stakeholders.

**5C.10.** Communicates effectively throughout consultation processes.

**5C.11.** Documents the scope and effectiveness of consultation activities.

**5C.12.** Maintains confidentiality as appropriate, ethically, and legally required throughout the consultation process.

## Additional Competencies for the Advanced Public Health Nurse

In addition to the competencies for the PHN, the APHN:

**5C.13A.** Provides expert consultation within and across systems and with individuals, families, groups, populations, and communities.

**5C.14A.** Provides professional expertise as requested, contracted, and appropriate during consultation processes.

**5C.15A.** Facilitates the identification and framing of problems and issues for consideration, exploration, and deliberation.

**5C.16A.** Provides expert testimony at the local, state, and federal levels on public health issues, policies, programs, and services for at-risk and vulnerable populations.

**5C.17A.** Synthesizes data from local, state, federal, and credible sources in consultation with the community and other stakeholders.

**5C.18A.** Generates proposals and reports in support of needed changes and decisions arising from consultation and as agreed upon or contracted.

**5C.19A.** Facilitates stakeholder consideration of issues and problems from multiple and diverse perspectives (e.g., theoretical, ethical, practical, and legal).

**5C.20A.** Acknowledges the limits and boundaries of the consulting role and constraints, such as history, traditions, alliances, allegiances, or policies, that may influence decision-making.

**5C.21A.** Raises creative suggestions and questions that may challenge the status quo and lay the groundwork for change.

**5C.22A.** Avoids premature closure and rush to judgment during consultation processes.

**5C.23A.** Conveys flexible, systematic, and meta-systematic reasoning throughout consultation.

**5C.24A.** Nurtures stakeholder creativity and risk taking with thinking.

**5C.25A.** Fosters openness and comfort with uncertainty and ambiguity during tentative and iterative processes.

**5C.26A.** Guides processes for decision-making, including negotiating, consensus building, and democratic or consensus decision-making.

**5C.27A.** Communicates understanding of the ethical nature of interdependent relationships and the value of common aims.

**5C.28A.** Seeks to understand the structure and functioning of the community, system, organization, or entity and how these may influence change.

**5C.29A.** Maximizes the inclusion of input from the communities served when developing public health policies, programs, and services.

**5C.30A.** Demonstrates how to gather information, analyze data and evidence, and practically apply theoretical and ethical knowledge in decision-making during consultation.

**5C.31A.** Balances facilitation, participation, and observation during consultation processes.

# STANDARD 5D. POLICY AND REGULATORY ACTIVITIES

The PHN participates in policy and regulatory activities related to health.

## Competencies
The PHN:

**5D.1.** Analyzes one's own knowledge of public health laws, regulations, and policies.

**5D.2.** Demonstrates knowledge of public health laws, regulations, and policies.

**5D.3.** Describes the structure, function, and jurisdictional authority of the organizational units within local, tribal, state, and federal public health agencies and their impact on individuals, families, and groups within a population.

**5D.4.** Educates affected populations on the development and application of relevant laws, regulations, and policies.

**5D.5.** Applies public health policies, programs, and resources in partnership with the population of interest.

**5D.6.** Promotes compliance with public health laws, regulations, and policies.

**5D.7.** Contributes to the intersectoral team to implement public health regulatory requirements, such as case identification, mandatory reporting, and program management.

**5D.8.** Contributes to emergency preparedness and response efforts, including the receipt and use of the strategic national stockpile.

## Additional Competencies for the Advanced Public Health Nurse
In addition to the competencies for the PHN, the APHN:

**5D.9A.** Designs public health programs and services consistent with public health laws, regulations, and policies.

**5D.10A.** Participates in all aspects of the policy process.

**5D.11A.** Develops partnerships with communities and agencies within the federal, state, tribal, and local levels of government that have authority over public health situations, such as emergency preparedness.

**5D.12A.** Designs compliance and reporting systems related to laws, regulations, and policies with other professionals.

**5D.13A.** Monitors compliance and reporting systems for quality and appropriate use of resources.

**5D.14A.** Analyzes data for reports for public health officials and other decision makers as required by laws, regulations, and policies.

**5D.15A.** Analyzes the impact of public health laws and regulations at the programmatic and organizational levels.

**5D.16A.** Ensures compliance with public health laws and regulations in the planning, implementation, and evaluation of community/population-based health services.

**5D.17A.** Participates in establishing, developing, implementing, and evaluating policy and regulatory activities.

# STANDARD 6. EVALUATION

The PHN evaluates progress toward attainment of goals and outcomes.

## Competencies
The PHN:

**6.1.** Conducts systematic, and ongoing, evaluations of programs and services in relation to the recommended program plan and indicated timeline.

**6.2.** Contributes to the evaluation plan for health promotion and health teaching programs and services.

**6.3.** Applies epidemiological and scientific methods to determine the effectiveness of PH nursing interventions.

**6.4.** Uses information technology to measure outcomes.

**6.5.** Uses multiple SDOH to evaluate outcomes of programs.

**6.6.** Uses ongoing assessment data to identify gaps and redundancies and to revise plans, interventions, and activities.

**6.7.** Collaborates with the target population and other key stakeholders involved in the evaluation process.

**6.8.** Gathers input from stakeholders when evaluating coordinated public health care service delivery.

**6.9.** Participates in evaluation by monitoring and ensuring appropriate use of programs and services to minimize unnecessary burden on the population.

**6.10.** Evaluates efficiency and effectiveness of community resources and associated programs in achieving population health outcomes.

**6.11.** Evaluates the effectiveness of CE strategies.

**6.12.** Disseminates the evaluation results to the population and other stakeholders.

**6.13.** Documents the results of the evaluation, including changes or recommendations to enhance the effectiveness of programs, services, and interventions.

## Additional Competencies for the Advanced Public Health Nurse

In addition to the competencies for the PHN, the APHN:

**6.14A.** Collaborates with the community and other relevant stakeholders in evaluations.

**6.15A.** Uses formal and informal networks when evaluating expected outcomes.

**6.16A.** Designs an evaluation plan with other public health experts and key stakeholders.

**6.17A.** Adapts the evaluation plan while considering policies, programs, or services.

**6.18A.** Uses evidence-based tools and epidemiologic data to evaluate program plans while considering SDOH within communities.

**6.19A.** Evaluates the accuracy of the population health assessment, the needs or problems, and the effectiveness of the plan for meeting expected and unexpected outcomes.

**6.20A.** Synthesizes the results of the evaluation and its impact on the program planning for populations, organizations, and stakeholder groups.

**6.21A.** Evaluates progress toward achieving national, state, and local health goals and objectives.

**6.22A.** Differentiates actual and expected system-level outcomes during program evaluation.

**6.23A.** Differentiates actual system-level intervention outcomes from expected outcomes.

**6.24A.** Evaluates efficiency and effectiveness of community resources and associated programs in achieving population health outcomes.

**6.25A.** Evaluates effectiveness of system-wide health care delivery guidelines, processes, and structures in efforts to promote equity and structural justice.

**6.26A.** Uses the results of evaluation analyses to recommend or make changes in policy, procedure, program, or services.

**6.27A.** Uses evaluation results of population-focused programs at the organizational level for quality, effectiveness, efficiency, safety, and sustainability.

# Standards of Professional Performance

## STANDARD 7. ETHICS

The PHN practices ethically.

## Competencies

The PHN:

**7.1.** Incorporates ANA's *Code of Ethics for Nurses with Interpretive Statements* (2015a) and the American Public Health Association's *Public Health Code of Ethics* (2019) in all practice areas.

**7.2.** Demonstrates how to apply ethics in PH nursing practice.

**7.3.** Practices with respect for the inherent dignity, worth, and unique attributes of persons and communities.

**7.4.** Promotes the protection of health and safety for all.

**7.5.** Protects autonomy, beliefs, dignity, values, and rights of the individual, family, group, community, or population.

**7.6.** Challenges public health practices that jeopardize health and safety.

**7.7.** Reports activities that are inconsistent with accepted standards of practice.

**7.8.** Applies ethical, legal, and policy guidelines and principles when collecting, maintaining, using, and disseminating data and information.

**7.9.** Collaborates with the public, other health professionals, legislators, policy leaders, and community decision makers to protect human rights, promote equity, and reduce health disparities.

**7.10.** Articulates nursing values to maintain the integrity of the nursing profession.

**7.11.** Integrates principles of social justice into practice.

**7.12.** Addresses the impact of discrimination, marginalization, and oppression on populations.

**7.13.** Maintains professional relationships and boundaries with individuals, families, and groups.

**7.14.** Participates in evidence-based training and ethical learning experiences.

**7.15.** Supports colleagues and others as they apply ethics to personal and professional situations and challenges.

## Additional Competencies for the Advanced Public Health Nurse
In addition to the competencies for the PHN, the APHN:

**7.16A.** Demonstrates the ability to mentor others in ethical decision-making.

**7.17A.** Partners with multisector teams to address ethical benefits, outcomes, and risks of policies, programs, and services.

**7.18A.** Creates policies, processes, and systems within the organization to maintain professional practice standards and ethics.

# STANDARD 8. RESPECTFUL AND EQUITABLE PRACTICE

The PHN practices with cultural sensitivity, humility, and safety and in a manner that is congruent with principles of cultural diversity, inclusion, and equity.

## Competencies
The PHN:

**8.1.** Applies cultural diversity, inclusion, and equity principles in PH nursing practice.

**8.2.** Demonstrates respect, equity, and empathy as well as cultural humility and safety in interactions with others.

**8.3.** Respects consumer decisions without bias.

**8.4.** Engages in life-long learning and self-reflection regarding one's own values, beliefs, cultural heritage, worldview, personal attitudes, and implicit biases.

**8.5.** Participates in life-long learning to understand cultural preferences, worldview, choices, and decision-making processes of diverse populations and stakeholders.

**8.6.** Applies knowledge of differences in health beliefs, practices, and communication patterns without assigning value to the differences in all nursing practice activities.

**8.7.** Addresses the effects and impact of discrimination and oppression on practice within and among diverse groups.

**8.8.** Uses appropriate skills and tools for the culture, literacy, and language of the population served.

**8.9.** Communicates with appropriate language and behaviors, including the use of certified interpreters and translators in accordance with population and stakeholder preferences.

**8.10.** Serves as a role model and educator for cultural humility, cultural safety, and the recognition and appreciation of diversity, equity, and inclusivity.

**8.11.** Identifies the culturally specific meaning of interactions, terms, and content.

**8.12.** Advocates for policies that promote health, prevent harm, and advance equity among culturally diverse, underserved, and underrepresented populations.

**8.13.** Promotes equity in all aspects of health, public health, and health care.

**8.14.** Advances organizational and public policies, programs, services, and practices that reflect respect, equity, and values for diversity and inclusion.

**8.15.** Promotes equal access to services, tests, interventions, health promotion, health education programs, and enrollment in research to promote health equity.

**8.16.** Uses data, evidence, and research about cultures to inform practice when working with diverse populations.

**8.17.** Applies knowledge of state and federal laws, regulations, and policies that support cultural congruence and safety in practice.

## Additional Competencies for the Advanced Public Health Nurse

In addition to the competencies for the PHN, the APHN:

**8.18A.** Engages populations, key stakeholders, and others in designing, establishing, and maintaining internal and external cross-cultural partnerships.

**8.19A.** Conducts research and quality improvement initiatives to improve health, public health, health care, and health outcomes for culturally diverse, underserved and/or marginalized populations.

**8.20A.** Develops recruitment and retention strategies to achieve a multicultural public health workforce.

**8.21A.** Promotes shared decision-making solutions in planning, implementing, and evaluating processes when the populations' cultural preferences, norms, and expectations may create incompatibility with evidence-based practice.

**8.22A.** Uses evaluation skills to ensure that tools, instruments, and services are acceptable and appropriate for culturally diverse populations.

**8.23A.** Advances organizational policies, programs, services, and practices that reflect respect, cultural humility, cultural safety, and values for diversity, equity, and inclusion.

**8.24A.** Leads interprofessional teams to identify the cultural, language, and health literacy needs of populations.

**8.25A.** Advocates for policies and practices in the workplace that promote a culture of diversity, equity, and inclusion.

**8.26A.** Advocates for policy, system, and environmental changes that advance equity for diverse populations.

# STANDARD 9. COMMUNICATION

The PHN communicates effectively in a variety of formats in all areas of practice.

## Competencies

The PHN:

**9.1.** Assesses one's own communication skills and effectiveness.

**9.2.** Seeks continuous improvement of individual communication styles using evidence-based communication principles.

**9.3.** Incorporates evidence-based communication techniques, including collaborative skills, negotiation, and conflict resolution.

**9.4.** Assesses communication format preferences of individuals, families, groups, communities, populations, and colleagues.

**9.5.** Integrates health literacy principles into all communications.

**9.6.** Implements evidence-based communication strategies or promising practices from across disciplines to promote health.

**9.7.** Translates information across intersectoral partners to ensure effective communication.

**9.8.** Employs a variety of methods and technologies to disseminate information widely.

**9.9.** Employs best practice communication methods to accommodate persons with special needs.

**9.10.** Documents communication to promote continuity of care, accountability in practice, and compliance with regulatory requirements.

**9.11.** Communicates observations and concerns to promote safety.

**9.12.** Incorporates appropriate strategies and information when effectively communicating about assessments, plans, interventions, evaluations, results, programs, and services.

**9.13.** Incorporates a continuous quality improvement process to advance communications.

**9.14.** Contributes a PH nursing perspective in discussions with the interprofessional team and intersectoral partners.

**9.15.** Communicates in a timely, legal, and ethical manner.

**9.16.** Demonstrates system-level critical thinking and complex decision-making skills when communicating with others.

**9.17.** Describes the implications of public health programs and policies to all stakeholders.

**9.18.** Models effective communication and presentations of the benefits, outcomes, and risks of policies, programs, services, and related decisions that affect the delivery of health-related information to relevant stakeholders.

## Additional Competencies for the Advanced Public Health Nurse

In addition to the competencies for the PHN, the APHN:

**9.19A.** Ensures that health literacy principles are integrated into internal and external organizational communications.

**9.20A.** Employs system-level approaches to disseminate public health information widely.

**9.21A.** Communicates decisions at the systems level, using a variety of communication modes.

**9.22A.** Mentors others in presentation and dissemination skills.

**9.23A.** Promotes compliance with public health laws and regulations in all communication.

**9.24A.** Ensures that organizational policies, processes, and systems support quality communication.

# STANDARD 10. COLLABORATION

The PHN collaborates with the population and others in the conduct of nursing practice.

## Competencies

The PHN:

**10.1.** Partners with stakeholders to navigate population-focused health concerns and effect change in public health policies, programs, and services.

**10.2.** Engages with formal and informal relational networks among community organizations and systems conducive to improving health.

**10.3.** Recruits relevant stakeholders to address public health issues.

**10.4.** Functions effectively with key stakeholders in activities that facilitate community involvement and delivery of services.

**10.5.** Promotes a culture of health as a shared value through CE.

**10.6.** Participates in stakeholder meetings to identify a shared vision, values, and principles for community action.

**10.7.** Builds stakeholder capacity to advocate for health issues.

**10.8.** Engages in teamwork and team-building processes to facilitate the development of interprofessional teams and workgroups.

**10.9.** Contributes as an interprofessional team member in developing organizational plans while ensuring compliance with established policies and program implementation guidelines.

**10.10.** Documents actions related to policies, programs, and services that indicate collaboration with populations and with others.

## Additional Competencies for the Advanced Public Health Nurse

In addition to the competencies for the PHN, the APHN:

**10.11A.** Forms partnerships with local, state, regional, and national organizations to address and sustain public health policies, programs, and services.

**10.12A.** Organizes stakeholders required to create community groups and coalitions to address public health issues affecting population health.

**10.13A.** Creates strategies that enhance collaboration within and across systems and organizations to address population health issues.

**10.14A.** Creates internal and external organizational relationships, processes, and system improvements to enhance the health of populations.

**10.15A.** Forms alliances across public and private health care systems that advance population health, equity, and well-being.

**10.16A.** Uses systems that ensure quality, collaboration, and coordination in the delivery of essential public health services.

**10.17A.** Builds functional capabilities of public health emergency preparedness across community sectors.

**10.18A.** Maximizes community partnerships that support clean, sustainable water and land, sanitation, food, air, and energy quality of the community.

**10.19A.** Influences policies, programs, and resources within and between organizations and systems that improve community and population well-being and health equity.

**10.20A.** Works in collaboration with intersectoral community partners to disseminate assessments, plans, and evaluations of public health services.

**10.21A.** Leads in establishing, improving, and sustaining collaborative relationships to promote population health.

**10.22A.** Appraises the effectiveness of CE and collaborative strategies on public health policies, programs, services, and resources.

**10.23A.** Documents communication, rationales for changes, and collaborative discussions related to public health policies, programs, and services to improve population outcomes.

# STANDARD 11. LEADERSHIP

The PHN leads within the professional practice setting and the profession.

## Competencies

The PHN:

**11.1.** Identifies internal and external factors affecting PH nursing practice and opportunities for interprofessional collaboration.

**11.2.** Acts in accordance with vision, mission, and organizational goals to improve the health of individuals, families, communities, or populations.

**11.3.** Facilitates development of organizational plans to implement programs and policies.

**11.4.** Facilitates development of interprofessional teams and workgroups.

**11.5.** Participates in teams to promote compliance with organizational policies.

**11.6.** Treats colleagues with respect, trust, and dignity.

**11.7.** Mentors colleagues in the acquisition of clinical knowledge, skills, abilities, and judgment.

**11.8.** Demonstrates ability to manage conflict in public health practice settings.

**11.9.** Participates in professional organizations relevant to their practice.

**11.10.** Identifies organizational and systems factors that affect PH nursing practice.

**11.11.** Seeks ways to advance the profession of nursing and the PH nursing specialty.

**11.12.** Articulates nursing and public health knowledge and skills to the interprofessional team, administrators, educators, policymakers, and appropriate intersectoral partners.

**11.13.** Participates in efforts to influence health care policy to increase access to care, improve quality of care, and ensure ethical and equitable provision of care.

## Additional Competencies for the Advanced Public Health Nurse

In addition to the competencies for the PHN, the APHN:

**11.14A.** Influences decision-making bodies to improve the professional practice environment and health outcomes.

**11.15A.** Provides direction to enhance the effectiveness of the interprofessional team.

**11.16A.** Promotes advanced PH nursing by interpreting its role for populations, partners, policymakers, and others.

**11.17A.** Models expert practice to intersectoral team members, interprofessional colleagues, and others.

**11.18A.** Mentors colleagues for the advancement of PH nursing practice and the nursing profession.

**11.19A.** Capitalizes on opportunities to mentor, advise, coach, and develop colleagues and other members of the public health workforce.

**11.20A.** Evaluates new approaches to public health practice that integrate organizational and systems thinking.

**11.21A.** Ensures that nursing is represented in interprofessional decision-making bodies.

**11.22A.** Organizes decision-making bodies to include relevant interprofessional representation.

**11.23A.** Functions as chief PHN strategist, ensuring that all relevant partners work in collaboration to drive prevention initiatives.

# STANDARD 12. EDUCATION

The PHN seeks knowledge and competence that reflect current nursing practice and promote futuristic thinking.

## Competencies
The PHN:

**12.1.** Identifies learning needs based on nursing and public health knowledge, the various roles the PHN may assume, and the changing needs of the population.

**12.2.** Uses individual, team, and organizational learning opportunities for personal and professional development as a PHN.

**12.3.** Seeks formal and independent learning experiences to develop and maintain competence, skills, and knowledge related to population health.

**12.4.** Shares educational findings, experiences, and ideas with peers.

**12.5.** Models personal commitment to lifelong learning, professional development, and advocacy.

**12.6.** Mentors nurses new to their roles to ensure their success.

**12.7.** Maintains professional records that provide evidence of competence and lifelong learning.

## Additional Competencies for the Advanced Public Health Nurse
In addition to the competencies for the PHN, the APHN:

**12.8A.** Facilitates a work environment supportive of ongoing professional development.

**12.9A.** Fosters the development of a personal commitment to lifelong learning, professional development, and advocacy.

**12.10A.** Uses intersectoral and multisystem collaboration to assess, evaluate, and analyze PHNs' continuing professional development needs.

# STANDARD 13. EVIDENCE-BASED PRACTICE AND RESEARCH

The PHN integrates evidence and research findings into practice.

## Competencies

The PHN:

**13.1.** Regularly evaluates research and other evidence for its relevance and applicability in PH nursing.

**13.2.** Uses the best available evidence, including PH nursing and public health research findings, to guide practice, policy, and service delivery decisions.

**13.3.** Uses evidence-based practice to meet core public health functions and the 10 essential public health services.

**13.4.** Participates in the formulation of EBP through ethical research activities.

**13.5.** Integrates evidence-based strategies or promising practices from across disciplines to promote health.

**13.6.** Facilitates involvement of communities, populations, organizations, and other stakeholder groups in participatory research processes.

**13.7.** Shares research activities and findings with colleagues and community stakeholders.

**13.8.** Contributes effectively as a member of a CBPR team.

## Additional Competencies for the Advanced Public Health Nurse

In addition to the competencies for the PHN, the APHN:

**13.9A.** Advocates for access to health sciences literature to enable EBP.

**13.10A.** Uses public health and nursing science in practice at community and population levels.

**13.11A.** Synthesizes evidence to inform current practice to improve health care systems, population health, and associated outcomes.

**13.12A.** Integrates evidence with professional expertise and community/ stakeholder preferences and values to improve health care systems and population health.

**13.13A.** Guides the integration of relevant research and evidence into PH nursing practice.

**13.14A.** Promotes research and scientific inquiry in the practice environment.

**13.15A.** Contributes to nursing, public health, and social science knowledge by conducting research.

**13.16A.** Ethically conducts research to improve the health of the public.

**13.17A.** Evaluates evidence-based data, programs, and strategies or promising practices to support strategies that address scientific, political, ethical, and social public health issues.

**13.18A.** Maximizes organizational effectiveness by translating research into practice.

**13.19A.** Addresses limitations of research findings with academic partners, internal and external stakeholders, and other public health professionals.

**13.20A.** Supports research across disciplines related to public health priorities and population-level interventions.

**13.21A.** Incorporates CBPR and other methods to evaluate the effectiveness of population-level health strategies, services, and programs for reducing the impact of SDOH.

**13.22A.** Ensures that the design, conduct, and dissemination of research is in partnership with populations and stakeholders to improve public health services and health outcomes for culturally diverse populations.

**13.23A.** Creates partnerships with academic and other organizations to expand the public health science base and disseminate research findings.

**13.24A.** Disseminates current evidence through presentations, publications, consultations, and use of media.

# STANDARD 14. QUALITY OF PRACTICE

The PHN contributes to quality nursing practice.

## Competencies

The PHN:

**14.1.** Participates in quality improvement teams.

**14.2.** Uses quality indicators and core measures to identify and address opportunities for improvement in services.

**14.3.** Implements operational procedures for public health programs and services.

**14.4.** Identifies data to evaluate services for individuals, families, and groups.

**14.5.** Contributes to the evaluation plan for PH nursing services.

**14.6.** Modifies PH nursing services based on reported evaluation results.

**14.7.** Participates in the implementation of the organization's performance management system.

**14.8.** Uses self-reflection to identify one's performance management improvement in the organization's performance management system.

**14.9.** Lists contributions to the organization's performance management system.

**14.10.** Identifies organizational initiatives that provide opportunities to improve the quality of PH nursing practice.

**14.11.** Provides feedback on the organization's mission and vision and the impact on individuals, families, and groups.

**14.12.** Seeks feedback on the organization's mission and vision and the impact on individuals, families, and groups.

## Additional Competencies for the Advanced Public Health Nurse

In addition to the competencies for the PHN, the APHN:

**14.13A.** Uses data and information to improve organizational processes and performance.

**14.14A.** Applies ethical, legal, and policy guidelines and principles in the collection, maintenance, use, and dissemination of data and information.

**14.15A.** Designs systems to measure, report, and improve quality of services and organizational performance.

# STANDARD 15. PROFESSIONAL PRACTICE APPRAISAL

The PHN evaluates personal nursing practice in relation to professional practice standards, guidelines, and relevant law.

## Competencies
The PHN:

**15.1.** Identifies one's own strengths in PH nursing practice and areas in which professional development could be beneficial.

**15.2.** Provides evidence for decisions and actions taken in PH nursing practice during evaluation processes.

**15.3.** Obtains feedback regarding one's own PH nursing practice from community members, professional colleagues, and others.

**15.4.** Takes action to achieve professional goals identified through formal and informal evaluation processes.

**15.5.** Evaluates the impact of standards, laws, certification, and licensure requirements on one's own PH nursing practice.

**15.6.** Demonstrates the ability to support civility, diversity, inclusion, and equity in collaborative environments.

**15.7.** Demonstrates active engagement of marginalized and disadvantaged groups and populations in decision-making that affects their well-being.

**15.8.** Demonstrates openness to input from individuals, groups, populations, and relevant stakeholders through the ability to integrate such input in public health programs and services.

**15.9.** Offers feedback to peers regarding PH nursing practice or role performance.

**15.10.** Reflects on one's own cultural awareness and cultural sensitivity in practice with diverse stakeholders.

**15.11.** Evaluates one's own implementation of culturally and age-appropriate nursing practice.

**15.12.** Demonstrates ethical awareness and ethical sensitivity when interacting with diverse stakeholders.

**15.13.** Adapts the delivery of PH nursing in consideration of changes in the public health system and the larger social, political, and economic environment.

## Additional Competencies for the Advanced Public Health Nurse

In addition to the competencies for the PHN, the APHN:

**15.14A.** Participates in a formal and systematic process when seeking feedback on PH nursing practice from professional colleagues, community members, and professional stakeholders.

**15.15A.** Analyzes one's own PH nursing practice in relation to certification and licensure requirements.

**15.16A.** Evaluates one's own effectiveness in collaborative relationships and partnerships within and across organizations and systems

**15.17A.** Promotes diversity, equity, and inclusion through the ongoing evaluation of organizational, agency, or systems processes, policies, and structures.

**15.18A.** Reinforces the values of diversity, civility, inclusion, and equity in all environments.

**15.19A.** Demonstrates knowledge of best practices, trends, and innovations in nursing and public health.

# STANDARD 16. RESOURCE UTILIZATION

The PHN uses appropriate resources to plan and provide nursing and public health services that are safe, effective, and financially responsible.

## Competencies
The PHN:

**16.1.** Identifies the individual, community, and population assets and available resources through data collection and stakeholder input.

**16.2.** Uses an ecological perspective and epidemiological data to identify the population's needs, potential for harm, complexity, and desired outcomes when considering resource allocation.

**16.3.** Engages formal and informal relational networks among community organizations and systems to improve health.

**16.4.** Incorporates evidence-based strategies or promising practices related to resource utilization to promote health in communities and populations.

**16.5.** Identifies evidence of the effectiveness of CE strategies.

**16.6.** Uses assets and resources within government, private, and nonprofit sectors to promote health and deliver services.

**16.7.** Advocates for resources, including human resources and technology, to enhance nursing practice, programs, and services.

**16.8.** Engages quality-improvement teams to promote positive interaction among populations, providers, technology, and other resources.

**16.9.** Assists representatives of specific populations and other stakeholders in identifying and securing appropriate and available services and resources to address health-related needs.

**16.10.** Provides information about the options, costs, risks, and benefits of policies, programs, and services.

**16.11.** Explains the impact and implications of budget constraints on delivering PH nursing services.

**16.12.** Identifies PH nursing services and programmatic needs to inform budget priorities.

**16.13.** Provides input into the fiscal and narrative components of proposals for funding from external sources.

**16.14.** Demonstrates knowledge of funding streams and the ability to contribute to grant writing that supports public health programs.

## Additional Competencies for the Advanced Public Health Nurse

In addition to the competencies for the PHN, the APHN:

**16.15A.** Uses the expertise of an interprofessional team to develop plans, design strategies, and implement programs.

**16.16A.** Creates organizational policies to elicit input from diverse partners.

**16.17A.** Utilizes organizational and community resources to formulate intersectoral plans for policies, programs, and services.

**16.18A.** Establishes programmatic budget priorities based on program outcomes, stakeholders, cost analysis, and financial information.

**16.19A.** Demonstrates fiscal responsibility and integrity in resource utilization.

**16.20A.** Formulates innovative approaches to address community and public health concerns.

**16.21A.** Designs implementation and evaluation strategies for population-focused programs to demonstrate cost-effectiveness and cost-benefit.

# STANDARD 17. ENVIRONMENTAL HEALTH, PLANETARY HEALTH, AND ENVIRONMENTAL JUSTICE

The PHN practices in an environmentally safe, fair, and just manner.

## Competencies

The PHN:

**17.1.** Recognizes the environment as a determinant of health that affects health equity and well-being.

**17.2.** Incorporates environmental context in applying nursing, public health, and social sciences to public health decision-making.

**17.3.** Ensures that community health assessments use an ecological perspective to identify and assess health risks from environmental hazards (e.g., chemical, biological, radiological, nuclear, explosive, physical, and/or psychosocial.)

**17.4.** Addresses the connections among person, environment, and health when applying the nursing process.

**17.5.** Recognizes the interplay among the environment, human actions, and genomics on human health and illness.

**17.6.** Identifies actual and potential policy outcomes relevant to environmental health and environmental justice.

**17.7.** Engages partners, stakeholders, and the community in identifying and addressing environmental health risks.

**17.8.** Communicates environmental health risks and exposure reduction strategies to promote and protect health and well-being.

**17.9.** Uses scientific evidence and the Precautionary Principle to guide decision-making that protects planetary, human, and environmental health and minimizes harm from environmental hazards, even when evidence of potential harm is indeterminate.

**17.10.** Participates in developing and implementing strategies to promote healthy homes, workplaces, schools, and communities.

**17.11.** Advocates for the judicious and appropriate use and environmentally safe disposal of products in the home, workplace, and community.

**17.12.** Advocates for implementation of environmental principles in PH nursing practice and public health.

**17.13.** Incorporates learning needs related to environmental health, planetary health, and environmental justice in one's own professional development plan.

**17.14.** Uses individual, team, and organizational learning opportunities to maintain knowledge of current environmental health, planetary health, and environmental justice issues, concepts, and trends relevant to all levels of population-focused prevention, including emergency preparedness.

## Additional Competencies for the Advanced Public Health Nurse

In addition to the competencies for the PHN, the APHN:

**17.15A.** Analyzes the impacts of social, political, and economic influences on human and environmental health at local, regional, and global levels.

**17.16A.** Supports nurses in advocating for and implementing principles of planetary health and environmental health programs with community and multidisciplinary partners to promote environmental justice and protect safe and healthy environments.

**17.17A.** Uses community assessment data and plans to develop policies, recommendations, and programs that address threats and prevent hazards to people and the natural environment.

**17.18A.** Promotes collaboration among PH nursing and relevant stakeholders to promote and advocate for environmentally healthy communities, planetary health, and environmental justice.

**17.19A.** Contributes to research addressing the connections between the environment, its conditions, and health status.

# STANDARD 18. ADVOCACY

The PHN advocates for the protection of health, safety, and the rights of communities and populations.

## Competencies

The PHN:

**18.1.** Identifies barriers to well-being and health.

**18.2.** Advocates for planning, implementing, and evaluating programs, policies, and services to improve health.

**18.3.** Articulates the need for culturally appropriate resources to enhance PH nursing services.

**18.4.** Identifies opportunities for individuals, families, communities, and populations to link with advocacy organizations.

**18.5.** Demonstrates needed skills in advocating on behalf of individuals, families, communities, and populations.

**18.6.** Identifies evidenced-based advocacy strategies to address the needs of diverse and underserved populations.

**18.7.** Assists individuals, families, communities, populations, and stakeholders in developing skills for self-advocacy.

**18.8.** Models personal commitment to advocacy for the nursing profession and the public at large.

## Additional Competencies for the Advanced Public Health Nurse

In addition to the competencies for the PHN, the APHN:

**18.9A.** Engages with public representatives, decision makers, advocacy groups, and consumer alliances on behalf of individuals, families, communities, and populations.

**18.10A.** Collaborates with decision makers in advocating for public health policies, programs, and services to promote healthy populations and communities.

**18.11A.** Serves as an expert for peers, populations, providers, and other stakeholders in promoting public health policies.

**18.12A.** Provides expert testimony at the local, state, and federal levels on delivery of programs and services for at-risk populations.

**18.13A.** Develops advocacy strategies for safe, competent, compassionate, and ethical care to address diverse and underserved populations' needs.

**18.14A.** Leads advocacy efforts for public health policies, programs, and resources that enhance services to communities and populations.

**18.15A.** Leverages public health priorities that improve population health, affect health care systems, and enhance equity.

# Glossary

**Aggregates/groups**—Groups within the larger population identified by health professionals as having one or more common characteristics, such as a specific health condition; engaging in behaviors with the potential to negatively affect health; sharing a common risk factor or risk exposure; or experiencing an emerging health threat or risk.

**Anchor**—A reliable community leader, principal support person, mainstay.

**Care continuum**—A concept involving an integrated system of care that guides and tracks patients over time through a comprehensive array of health services spanning all levels of intensity of care.

**Community**—A set of people in interaction who may or may not share a sense of place or belonging and who act intentionally for a common purpose (e.g., live in a neighborhood, work at a given company, or share a common cultural or demographic characteristic, health condition, or threat to health).

**Community-based participatory research (CBPR)**—Focuses on establishing equitable partnerships, addressing a population's needs based in collaboration with them, and responding to what the community has identified as the primary issue.

**Cultural diversity**—The existence of a variety of cultural or ethnic groups within a society.

**Cultural humility**—A humble and respectful attitude toward individuals of other cultures that pushes one to challenge one's own cultural biases, realize that one cannot possibly know everything about other cultures, and approach learning about other cultures as a life-long goal and process.

**Cultural sensitivity**—The ability to be open and responsive to attitudes, feelings, or life circumstances of groups of people who share common distinctive aspects of racial, national, religious, linguistic, or cultural heritage.

**Culturally congruent practice**—Application of evidence-based nursing within the context of the preferred cultural values, beliefs, worldview, and practices of the health care consumer, community, and other stakeholders.

**Determinants of health**—The conditions in which people are born, grow, live, work, and age. They are shaped by the distribution of money, power, and resources at global, national, and local levels.

**Disparities**—"A noticeable and usually significant difference or dissimilarity" (Merriam-Webster, n.d.).

**Ecological model of health**—The interaction between, and interdependence of, factors within and across all levels of health.

**Ecological perspective**—A useful framework for understanding the range of factors that influence health and well-being. It is a model that can assist in providing a complete perspective of the factors that affect specific health behaviors, including the social determinants of health (SDOH).

**Equity**—The quality of being fair and impartial.

**Formative evaluation**—Ongoing evaluation and monitoring that shows whether a project/process is being implemented as planned and whether short- and mid-term indicators are moving in the direction desired, allowing for adaption of the plan to better achieve desired outcomes.

**Genomics**—The branch of molecular biology concerned with the structure, function, evolution, and mapping of genomes.

**Health equity**—"Health equity is defined as the absence of unfair and avoidable or remediable differences in health among population groups defined socially, economically, demographically or geographically" (WHO, n.d.).

**Intersectoral**—Action that involves several sectors of society—for instance action by the health, education, housing, and local government sectors to enhance community health.

**Planetary health**—A field in public health that is focused on characterizing the human health impacts of human-caused disruptions of Earth's natural systems (Planetary Health Alliance, n.d.).

"The concept of planetary health is based on the understanding that human health and human civilization depend on flourishing natural systems and the wise stewardship of those natural systems" (Whitmee et al., 2015). "Planetary health seeks to safeguard the health of present and future generations and promote intergenerational and intragenerational equity and justice" (Wabnitz et al., 2020).

**Political determinants of health**—The intersection of multiple and various factors driven by law and policy create conditions that can negatively influence the health of individuals and populations. Specific political determinants of health include voting, government, policies, politics, and policymaking. Each can systematically contribute to producing, sustaining, and exacerbating the inequalities that exist in society and contribute to health inequities.

**Population**—A collection of individuals in a geographically defined area (e.g., town, city, state, region, nation, or multinational region) or a group of individuals within the community (such as school students, workers in industry, or persons of similar age).

**Population health**—The health outcomes of a group of people, including the distribution of such outcomes within the group.

**Population health management**—Management of health outcomes of a clinical population enrolled in a discrete health care system that is held financially accountable.

**Precautionary principle**—The precautionary principle guides decision-making and acknowledges that, in the absence of sufficient scientific evidence, the appropriate action is caution and avoidance of unnecessary risk.

**Racism**—"Policies, behaviors, rules, etc. that result in a continued unfair advantage to some people and unfair or harmful treatment of others based on race." "Harmful or unfair things that people say, do, or think based on the belief that their own race makes them more intelligent, good, moral, etc. than people of other races" (Cambridge University, n.d.-a).

**Social betterment**—"Social betterment refers to the improvement of social conditions. Put differently, in the context of democratic society, social betterment refers to bringing about a state that would be considered as better than the state that existed before, as judged though deliberation and by public opinion" (Henry & Mark, 2003, p. 295).

**Social ecological model**—"The social ecological model (SEM) guides health promotion as well as illness prevention interventions. According to this model, health care and health-related behavior are a function of individual, interpersonal, organizational, community, and population factors" (Kulbok & Botchwey, 2016, p. 385).

**Social justice**—Social justice is the moral foundation of public health and health policy (Powers & Faden, 2006). Social justice aspires to prevent injustices from occurring. It is achieved by altering background conditions that lead to marginalization, exploitation, exclusion, powerlessness, and violence (Young, 1990). Social justice is achieved by correcting institutional and structural conditions that create injustices and inequalities and that disadvantage or harm vulnerable groups (Young, 2011). The aims of social justice are well-being and health equity (Powers & Faden, 2006).

**Structural racism**—"Laws, rules, or official policies in a society that result in and support a continued unfair advantage to some people and unfair or harmful treatment of others based on race" (Cambridge University, n.d.-b).

**Summative evaluation**—Evaluation typically completed after/at the term of the project/budget cycle to assess whether desired outcomes were achieved and how the outcomes were achieved (e.g., were the planned interventions and resources used, including documentation of the adaptation of the planned interventions and resources?).

**Systemic racism**—"Policies and practices that exist throughout a whole society or organization, and that result in and support a continued unfair advantage to some people and unfair or harmful treatment of others based on race" (Cambridge University, n.d.-c ).

**Well-being**—"[W]ell-being includes the presence of positive emotions and moods (e.g., contentment, happiness), the absence of negative emotions (e.g., depression, anxiety), satisfaction with life, fulfillment and positive functioning. In simple terms, well-being can be described as judging life positively and feeling good. For public health purposes, physical well-being (e.g., feeling very healthy and full of energy) is also viewed as critical to overall well-being" ( CDC, 2018, October 31).

# References

Abbott, L. S. (2014). Evaluation of nursing interventions designed to impact knowledge, behaviors, and health outcomes for rural African-Americans: An integrative review. *Public Health Nursing, 32*(5), 408–420.

Affordable Care Act (ACA). (2010). https://www.healthcare.gov/glossary/affordable-care-act/.

Agency for Healthcare Research and Quality (AHRQ). (2014). Care Coordination. https://www.ahrq.gov/ncepcr/care/coordination.html.

Alderwick, H., & Gottlieb, L. M. (2019). Meanings and misunderstandings: A social determinants of health lexicon for health care systems. *Milbank Quarterly, 97*(2), 407–419.

Alexander, G. (2020). Supporting food literacy among children and adolescents: Undergraduate students apply public health nursing principles in clinical practice. *Journal of Professional Nursing*, in press. https://www.sciencedirect.com/science/article/pii/S875572232030168X.

American Association of Colleges of Nursing (AACN). (2008). *The essentials of baccalaureate education for professional nursing practice.* https://www.aacnnursing.org/Portals/42/Publications/BaccEssentials08.pdf.

————. (2020). Personal communication.

American Nurses Association (ANA). (1973). *Standards of community health nursing practice.* Kansas City, MO: Author.

————. (1986). *Standards of community health nursing practice.* Kansas City, MO: Author.

————. (1999). *Scope and standards of public health nursing practice.* Washington, DC: Author.

————. (2007). *Public health nursing: Scope and standards of practice.* Silver Spring, MD: Author.

————. (2013). *Public health nursing: Scope and standards of practice, second edition.* Silver Spring, MD: Author.

————. (2014). *Professional Role Competence Position Statement.* Silver Spring, MD: Author. https://www.nursingworld.org/practice-policy/nursing-excellence/official-position-statements/id/professional-role-competence/.

————. (2015a). *Code of ethics for nurses with interpretive statements.* Silver Spring, MD: Author.

_____. (2015b). *Nursing: Scope and standards of practice, third edition*. Silver Spring, MD: Author.

_____. (2015c). *ANA position statement on incivility, bullying and workplace violence*. Silver Spring, MD: Author. https://www.nursingworld.org/practice-policy/nursing-excellence/official-position-statements/id/incivility-bullying-and-workplace-violence/.

_____. (2021). *Nursing: Scope and standards of practice, fourth edition*. Silver Spring, MD: Author.

American Nurses Credentialing Center (ANCC). (2020). Our certifications. https://www.nursingworld.org/our-certifications/.

American Public Health Association, Public Health Nursing Section. (2013). *The definition and practice of public health nursing*. Washington, DC: Author. https://www.apha.org/~/media/files/pdf/membergroups/phn/nursingdefinition.ashx.

American Public Health Association (APHA). (1996). *The definition and role of public health nursing*. Washington, DC: Author.

_____. (2019). *Public health code of ethics*. www.APHA.org.

Anderson, E. T., & McFarlane, J. M. (2019). *Community as partner: Theory and practice in nursing*. Philadelphia: Wolters Kluwer.

Association for Prevention Teaching and Research (APTR). (2020). *Clinical prevention and population health curricular framework*. http://www.teachpopulation-health.org/.

Association of Community Health Nursing Educators (ACHNE). (2010). *Essentials of baccalaureate nursing education for entry-level community/public health nursing*.

Baker, E. L., & Koplan, J. P. (2002). Strengthening the nation's public health infrastructure: Historic challenge, unprecedented opportunity. *Health Affairs, 21*(6), 15–27.

Baldwin, J. A., Johnson, J. L., & Benally, C. C. (2009). Building partnerships between indigenous communities and universities: Lessons learned in HIV/AIDS and substance abuse prevention research. *American Journal of Public Health, 99*(S1), S77–S82.

Baldwin, J. H., Conger, C. O., Abegglen, J. C., & Hill, E. M. (1998). Population-focused and community-based nursing—Moving toward clarification of concepts. *Public Health Nursing, 15*(1), 12–18.

Beauchamp, D. E. (2003). Public health as social justice. In R. Hofrichter (ed.), *Health and social justice: Politics, ideology, and inequity in the distribution of disease* (267–284). San Francisco, CA: Jossey-Bass.

Beck, A. J., & Boulton, M. L. (2016). The public health workforce in U.S, state and local health departments, 2012. *Public Health Report, Jan–Feb 131*(1), 145–152. doi:1 0.1177/003335491613100121.

Bekemeier, B., Grembowski, D., Yang, Y., & Herting, J. (2012). Leadership matters: Local health department clinician leaders and their relationship to decreasing health disparities. *Journal of Public Health Management and Practice, 18*(2), E1–E10. doi:10.1097/PHH.0b013e318242d4fc.

Bekemeier, B., Linderman, T., Kneipp, S., & Zahner, S. (2014). Updating the definition and role of public health nursing to advance and guide the specialty. *Public Health Nursing, 32*(1), 50–57.

Berwick, D. M., Nolan, T. W., & Whittington, J. (2008). The triple aim: Care, health, and cost. *Health Affairs, Millwood, 27*(3), 759–769.

Bigbee, J. L., Gehrke, P., & Otterness, N. (2009). Public health nurses in rural/ frontier one-nurse offices. *Rural Remote Health, Oct–Dec 9*(4): 1282.

Blackstone, A. (2012). Principles of sociological inquiry—Qualitative and quantitative methods. Saylor Foundation.

Bodenheimer, T., & Sinsky, C. (2014). From triple to quadruple aim: Care of the patient requires care of the provider. *Annals of Family Medicine, 12*(6), 573–576. https://doi.org/10.1370/afm.1713.

Brainard, A. M. (1995). *The evolution of public health nursing.* New York: Garland. (Original work published in 1922. Philadelphia: W. B. Saunders.)

Brandt, A. M. (2021). Pandemics and public health history. *American Journal of Public Health*, 111(3), 409–410.

Braveman, P. (2014). What are health disparities and health equity? We need to be clear. *Public Health Reports, 129* (Supplement 2), 5–8.

———. (2019). Swimming against the tide: Challenges in pursuing health equity today. *Academic Medicine, 94*(2), 170–171.

Braveman, P., Arkin, E., Orleans, T., Proctor, D., & Plough, A. (2017). What is health equity? Robert Wood Johnson Foundation. https://www.rwjf.org/en/ library/research/2017/05/what-is-health-equity-.html.

Braveman, P. A., Kumanyika, S., Fielding, J., LaVeist, T., Borrell, L. N., Manderscheid, R., & Troutman, A. (2011). Health disparities and health equity: The issue is justice. *American Journal of Public Health, 101*(81), S149–S155.

Bresnick, J. (2017). How do population health, public health, community health differ?https://healthitanalytics.com/news/how-do-population-health-public-health-community-health-differ.

Broussard, D. L., Wallace, M. E., Richardson, L., & Theall, K. P. (2020). Building governmental public health capacity to advance health equity: Conclusion based on an environmental scan of a local public health system, *Health Equity, 4*(1), 362–365. doi:10.1089/heq.2019.0025.

Buettner-Schmidt, K., & Lobo, M. (2011). Social justice: A concept analysis. *Journal of Advanced Nursing, 68*(4), 948–958. doi:10.1111/j.1365-2648.2011.05856.x.

Cambridge University. (n.d.-a). Racism. In *Cambridge Dictionary Online.* https://dictionary.cambridge.org/us/dictionary/english/racism.

Cambridge University. (n.d.-b). Structural racism. In *Cambridge Dictionary Online.* https://dictionary.cambridge.org/us/dictionary/english/structural-racism.

Cambridge University. (n.d.-c). Systemic racism. In *Cambridge Dictionary Online.* https://dictionary.cambridge.org/us/dictionary/english/systemic-racism.

Campinha-Bacote, J. (2002). The process of cultural competence in the delivery of healthcare services: A model of care. *Journal of Transcultural Nursing, 13,* 181–184.

Carabez, R., & Kim, J. E. (2019). PART I: The role of public health nursing in addressing health care needs of children in foster care. *Public Health Nursing, 36*(5), 702–708.

Carse, A. (1996). Facing up to moral perils: The virtues of care in bioethics. In S. Gordon, P. Benner, & N. Noddings (eds.), *Caregiving: Readings in knowledge, practice, ethics and politics* (83–110). Philadelphia: University of Pennsylvania Press.

Castle, B., Wendel, M., Kerr, J., Brooms D., & Rollins, A. (2019). Public health's approach to systemic racism: A systematic literature review. *Journal of Racial Ethnic Health Disparities, 6*(1), 27–36. doi:10.1007/s40615-018-0494-x.

Centers for Disease Control and Prevention (CDC). (n.d.-a) *Health Equity.* www.cdc.gov/chronicdisease/healthequity.

————. (n.d.-b) *Picture of America prevention.* https://www.cdc.gov/pictureofamerica/pdfs/picture_of_america_prevention.pdf.

————. (2011). *Principles of community engagement, second edition.* https://www.atsdr.cdc.gov/communityengagement/pdf/PCE_Report_508_FINAL.pdf.

————. (2018, October 31). Well-being concepts: *Why is well-being useful for public health?* https://www.cdc.gov/hrqol/wellbeing.htm#one.

————. (2020, March 18). *Ten essential services of public health.* https://www.cdc.gov/publichealthgateway/publichealthservices/essentialhealthservices.html.

————. (2019, December 19). *Frequently asked questions: What are social determinants of health?* https://www.cdc.gov/nchhstp/socialdeterminants/faq.html#what-are-social-determinants.

_____. (2020, August 3). *What is Epigenetics?* https://www.cdc.gov/genomics/disease/epigenetics.htm.

Center for Public Health Nursing Practice. (2003). *The nursing process applied to population-based public health nursing practice.* Minnesota Department of Health. https://www.health.state.mn.us/communities/practice/ta/phnconsultants/docs/0303phn_processapplication.pdf.

Chandra, A., Acosta, J. D., Carman, K. G., Dubowitz, T., Leviton, L., Martin, L. T., Miller, C., Nelson, C., Orleans, T., Tait, M., Trujillo, M., Towe, V. L., Yeung, D., & Plough, A. L. (2016). Building a national culture of health: Background, action, framework, measures, and next steps. *Rand Health Quarterly, 6*(2), 3. https://www.rand.org/pubs/research_reports/RR1199.html.

Chaudry, R. V. (2008). The precautionary principle, public health, and public health nursing. *Public Health Nursing, 25*(3), 261–268. https://doi.org/10.1111/j.1525-1446.2008.00703.x.

Chodorow, N. (1978). *The reproduction of mothering.* Berkeley: University of California Press.

Churchman, C. W. (1971). *The design of inquiring systems: Basic concepts of systems and organizations.* New York, NY: Basic Books.

Cohen, N. J., Brown, C. M., Alvarado-Ramy, F., Bair-Brake, H., Benenson, G. A., Chen, T., Demma, A. J., Holton, N. K., Kohl, K. S., Lee, A. W., McAdam, D., Pesik, N., Roohi, S., Smith, C. L., Waterman, S. H., & Cetron, M. S. l. (2016). Travel and border health measures to prevent the international spread of Ebola. *MMWR Supplement, 65*(Suppl-3), 57–67. http://dx.doi.org/10.15585/mmwr.su6503a9.

Community Preventive Services Task Force (CPSTF). 2020. https://www.thecommunityguide.org/about/about-community-guide.

Council on Linkages (CoL). (2017). Modified version of the core competencies for public health professionals. http://www.phf.org/resourcestools/PagesModified_Core_Competencies_for_Public_Health_Professionals.aspx.

Curtis, E., Jones, R., Tipene-Leach, D., Walker, C., Loring, B., Paine, S., & Papaarangi, R. (2019). Why cultural safety rather than cultural competency is required to achieve health equity: A literature review and recommended definition. *International Journal of Equity Health, 18*, 174. https://doi.org/10.1186/s12939-019-1082.

Danso, R. (2018). Cultural competence and cultural humility: A critical reflection on key cultural diversity concepts. *Journal of Social Work, 18*(4), 410–430. https://doi.org/10.117/1468017316654341.

Dawes, D. E. (2018). The future of health equity in America. Addressing the legal and political determinants of health. *Journal of Law, Medicine and Ethics, 46*, 838–840.

———. (2020). Health inequities: A look at the political determinants of health during the Covid-19 pandemic. *American Journal of Health Studies*, 35(2), 77–82.

DeSalvo, K. B., Wang, Y. C., Harris, A., Auerbach, J., Koo, D., & O'Carroll, P. (2017) Public health 3.0: A call to action for public health to meet the challenges of the 21st century. *Preventing Chronic Disease*, 14. https://www.cdc.gov/pcd/issues/2017/17_0017.htm.

Dickson E., & Lobo, M. L. (2018). Critical caring theory and public health nursing advocacy for comprehensive sexual health education. *Public Health Nursing, 35*, 78–84. https://doi.org/10.1111/phn.12369.

Dupin, C., Pinon, M., Jaggi, K., Teixera, C., Sagne, A., & Delicado, N. (2020). Public health nursing education viewed through the lens of superdiversity: A resource for global health. *BMC Nursing, 19*, 1–5.

Egede, L., & Walker, R. (2020). Structural racism, social risk factors, and Covid-19—A dangerous convergence for Black Americans. *New England Journal of Medicine, 383*. doi:10.1056/NEJMp2023616.

Edwards, K., Lund, C., Mitchell, S., & Andersson, N. (2008). Trust the process: Community-based researcher partnerships. *Pimatisiwin, 6*(2), 186–199.

Ervin, N., & Kulbok, P. A. (2018). *Advanced public and community health nursing practice: Population assessment, program planning and evaluation, second edition*. New York, NY: Springer Publishing Company. doi:10.1891/9780826138446.

Faden, R. R., Shebaya, S., & Siegel, A. W. (2019). Distinctive challenges of public health ethics. In A. C. Mastroianni, J. P. Kahn, & N.E. Kass (eds.), *The Oxford handbook of public health ethics* (12–20). New York, NY: Oxford University Press.

Farber Post, L., & Blustein, J. (2015). *Handbook for health care ethics committees, second edition*. Baltimore, MD: Johns Hopkins University Press.

Farmer, P. (2005). *Pathologies of power: Health, human rights, and the new war on the poor*. Berkeley: University of California Press.

Fisher-Borne, M., Cain, J. M., & Martin, S. (2015). From mastery to accountability: Cultural humility as an alternative to cultural competence. *Social Work Education: The International Journal, 34*(2), 165–181. https://doi.org/10.1080/02615479.2014.977244.

Fitzpatrick, M. L. (1975). *The National Organization for Public Health Nursing. 1912–1952: Development of a practice field*. New York: National League for Nursing.

Florez, J. (2007). Americans are losing sense of community. *Deseret News*. https://www.deseret.com/2007/5/7/20016893/john-florez-americans-are-losing-sense-of-community.

Fowler, M. D. (2020). Toward reclaiming our ethical heritage: Nursing ethics before bioethics. *OJIN: The Online Journal of Nursing, 25*(2).

Freire, P. (1970). *Pedagogy of the oppressed.* New York, NY: Seabury Press.

————. (1998). *Pedagogy of freedom: Ethics, democracy, and civic courage.* Lanham, MA: Rowman and Littlefield.

Frieden, T. (2010). A framework for public health action: The health impact pyramid. *American Journal of Public Health, 100*(4), 590–595.

Garey, D., & Hott, L. R. (Producers). (1988). *Sentimental women need not apply [Film].* Florentine Films.

Gilligan, C. (1982). *In a different voice: Psychological theory and women's development.* Cambridge, MA: Harvard University Press.

Gonzales, K., & Levitas, J. (2020). Cultural humility: Definition and example. https://study.com/academy/lesson/cultural-humility-definition-example.html.

Gorski, M., Polansky, P., & Swider, S. (2019). *Nursing education and the path to population health improvement.* Princeton, NJ: Future of Nursing Campaign for Action, Robert Wood Johnson Foundation, and AARP Foundation. https://campaignforaction.org/resource/nursing-education-and-the-path-to-population -health-improvement/.

Gostin, L. O., & Friedman, E. A. (2017). Global health: A pivotal moment of opportunity and peril. *Health Affairs, 36*(1), 159–165. doi:10.1377/hlthaff.2016.1492.

Guba, E. G., & Lincoln, Y. S. (1989). *Fourth generation evaluation.* Newbury Park, CA: Sage Publications.

Habermas, J. (1991). *Moral consciousness and communicative action.* Cambridge, MA: MIT Press.

Hagen, W. B., Hoover, S. M., & Morrow, S. L. (2018). A grounded theory of sexual minority women and transgender individuals' social justice activism. *Journal of Homosexuality, 65*(7), 833–859.

Hanlon, J. J., & Pickett, C. E. (eds). (1984). *Public health: Administration and practice, eighth edition.* St. Louis: Mosby.

Heffernan, M., Fromknecht, C. Q., McGowan, A. K., Blakely, C., & Oppenheimer, C. C. (2019). Healthy people for the 21st century: Understanding use of Healthy People 2020 as a web-based initiative. *Journal of Public Health Management and Practice, (25)*2: 121–127. doi:10.1097/PHH.0000000000000784.

Held, V. (2006). *The ethics of care: Personal, political and global.* New York, NY: Oxford University Press.

Henry, G. T., & Mark, M. M. (2003). Beyond use: Understanding evaluation's influence on attitudes and actions. *American Journal of Evaluation, 24*, 293–314.

Henry Street Consortium. (2017). Entry-level, population-based public health nursing competencies. St. Paul, MN: Author. www.henrystreetconsortium.org.

Hester, D. M., & Schonfeld, T. (eds.) (2016). *Guidance for healthcare ethics committees*. New York, NY: Cambridge University Press.

Institute for Healthcare Improvement (IHI). (2019). Triple aim for populations. http://www.ihi.org/Topics/TripleAim/Pages/default.aspx.

Institute of Medicine (IOM). (1988). *The future of public health*. Washington, DC: National Academies Press.

————. (2011). The future of nursing education. In *The Future of nursing: Leading change, advancing health*. Washington, DC: National Academies Press. doi:110.17226/12956.

Josiah Macy Jr. Foundation. (2016). Registered nurses: Partners in transforming primary care. http://macyfoundation.org/docs/macy_pubs/201609_Nursing_Conference_Exectuive_Summary_Final.pdf.

Keeys, M. (2021). The critical discussion of race and racism toward achieving equity in health policy. In M. P. Moss & J. M. Phillips, (eds). *Health equity and nursing achieving equity through policy, population health, and interprofessional collaboration*. Springer Publishing Company.

Kett, P. M. (2020). The individual focus of nursing research in breastfeeding: Perpetuating a neoliberal perspective. *Public Health Nursing, 37*, 281–286.

Kindig, D., & Stoddart, G. (2003). What is population health? *American Journal of Public Health, 93*(3), 380–383.

Kneipp, S. M., Kairalla, J. A., Lutz, B. J., Pereira, D., Hall, A. G., Flocks, F., Beeber, L., & Schwartz, T. (2011). Public health nursing case management for women receiving temporary assistance for needy families: A randomized controlled trial using community-based participatory research. *American Journal of Public Health, 101*(9), 1759–1768. doi:10.2105/AJPH.2011.300210.

Kneipp, S. M., Kairalla, J. A., & Sheely, A. L. (2013). A randomized controlled trial to improve health among women receiving welfare in the U.S.: The relationship between employment outcomes and the economic recession. *Social Science and Medicine, 80*, 130–140.

Kub, J., E., Kulbok, P. A., Miner, S., & Merrill, J. A. (2017). Increasing the capacity of public health nursing to strengthen the public health infrastructure and to promote and protect the health of communities and populations. *Nursing Outlook, 65*, 661–664.

Kulbok, P. A., & Botchwey, N. (2016). Building a culture of health through community health promotion. In M. Stanhope & J. Lancaster (eds.), *Public Health Nursing: Population-Centered Health Care in the Community* (377–394). St. Louis: Elsevier.

Kulbok, P. A., Thatcher, E., Park, E., & Meszaros, P. S. (2012). Evolving public health nursing roles: Focus on community participatory health promotion and prevention. *OJIN: The Online Journal of Issues in Nursing*, 17(2), Manuscript 1. https://doi.org/10.3912/OJIN.Vol17No02Man01.

LaChance, N. (2014). So long, neighbor. *U.S. News & World Report*. https://www.usnews.com/opinion/articles/2014/08/21/america-is-losing-its-sense-of-community-says-marc-dunkleman.

LaHolt, H., McLeod, K., Guillemin, M., Beddari, E., & Lorem, G. (2019). Ethical challenges experienced by public health nurses related to adolescents' use of visual technologies. *Nursing Ethics*, 26(6), 1822–1833.

Latham, S. (2016). Health care ethics committees and the law. In D. M. Hester & T. Schonfeld (eds.), *Guidance for healthcare ethics committees* (17–24). New York, NY: Cambridge University Press.

LeClair, J., Watts, T., & Zahner, S. (2021). Nursing strategies for environmental justice: A scoping review. *Public Health Nursing*, 38(2), 296–308.

Lee, L. M., & Zarowsky, C. (2015). Foundational values for public health. *Public Health Reviews*, 36, 2. doi:10.1186/s40985-015-0004-1.

Little, S., Swider, S. M., Andresen, K. M., Arcilla, D., Chaudry, R. V., Cooper, J. L., Decker, K. A., Edwards, L., Graham, J. C., Haushalter, A. R., Hensley, J. L., Koyama, K., Morton, J. L., Ouzts, K. N., Robinson, A., Saltzberg, C. W., Smith, C. M., & Weierbach, F. M. (2019). *Awareness and usage: Public health nursing: Scope and standards of practice and the Quad Council Coalition's 2018 community/public health nursing competencies*. Unpublished manuscript.

MacPherson, D. W., Gushulak, B. D., & MacDonalda, C. (2007). Health and foreign policy: Influences of migration and population mobility. *Bulletin of the World Health Organization*, 85(3), 200–206.

Mahony, D., & Jones, E. (2013). Social determinants of health in nursing education, research, and health policy. *Nursing Science Quarterly*, 26(3), 280–284.

Marckmann, G., Schmidt, H., Sofaer, N., & Strech, D. (2015). Putting public health ethics into practice: A systematic framework. *Frontiers in Public Health*, 3(23), 1–8.

Marion, L., Douglas, M., Lavin, M. A., Barr, N., Gazaway, S., Thomas, E., & Bickford, C. (2017). Implementing the new ANA standard 8: Culturally congruent practice. American Nurses Association. https://ojin.nursingworld.org/MainMenu Categories/ANAMarketplace/ANAPeriodicals/OJIN/TableofContents/

Vol-22-2017/No1-Jan-2017/Articles-Previous-Topics/Implementing-the-New-ANA-Standard-8.html.

Merriam-Webster. (n.d.). Disparity. In *Merriam-Webster.com dictionary*. https://www.merriam-webster.com/dictionary/disparity.

Minnesota Department of Health. (2019). *Public Health Interventions: Applications for Public Health Nursing Practice, second edition*. https://www.health.state.mn.us/communities/practice/research/phncouncil/wheel.html.

Monsen, K. A., Attleson, I. S., Ericson, K. J., Neely, C., Oftedahl, G., & Thorsen, D. R. (2015). Translation of obesity practice guidelines: Interprofessional perspectives regarding the impact of public health nurse system-level intervention. *Public Health Nursing, 32*(1), 34–42.

Monsen, K. A., Brandt, J. K., Brueshoff, B., Chi, C. L, Mathiason, M. A., Swenson, S. M., & Thorson, D. R. (2017). Social determinants and health disparities associated with outcomes of women of childbearing age receiving public health nurse home visiting services. *Journal of Obstetric, Gynecologic and Neonatal Nursing, 46*(2), 292–303.

Monsen, K. A., Fulkerson, J. A., Lytton, A. B., Taft, L. L., Schwichtenberg, L. D., & Martin, K. S. (2010). Comparing maternal child health problems and outcomes across public health nursing agencies. *Maternal and Child Health Journal, 14*(3), 412–421.

Monsen, K. A., Sanders, A. N., Yu, F., Radosevich, D. M., & Geppert, J. S. (2011). Family home visiting outcomes for mothers with and without intellectual disabilities. *Journal of Intellectual Disability Research, 55*(5), 484–499.

Murcia, S., & Lopez, L. (2016). The experience of nurses in care for culturally diverse families: A qualitative meta-synthese. Revista Latino-Americana de Enfermagem. University of Columbia. Bogota. *Epub* July 4, 2016. http://dx.doi.org/10.1590/1518-8345.1052.2718.

National Academies of Sciences, Engineering, and Medicine (NASEM). (2017). *Communities in action: Pathways to health equity*. Washington, DC: National Academies Press. https://doi.org/10.17226/24624.

———. (2021). *The Future of Nursing 2020–2030: Charting a Path to Achieve Health Equity*. http://www.nationalacademies.org/hmd/Activities/Workforce/futureofnursing2030.aspx.

National Board of Public Health Examiners (NBPHE). (n.d.). https://www.nbphe.org.

National Forum of State Workforce Centers. (2019). National workforce centers location map. https://nursingworkforcecenters.org/location-map/.

Noddings, N. (1984). *Caring: A Feminine Approach to Ethics and Moral Education*. Berkeley: University of California Press.

Office of Minority Health. (2001). *National standards for culturally and linguistically appropriate services in health care*. US Department of Health and Human Services. Washington, DC. https://minorityhealth.hhs.gov/assets/pdf/checked/finalreport.pdf.

Olsen, J. M., Horning, M. L, Thorson, D., & Monsen, K. A. (2018). Relationships between public health nurse-delivered physical activity interventions and client physical activity behavior. *Applied Nursing Research*, 40, 13–19.

Pittman, P. (2019). *Activating Nursing to Address Unmet Needs in the 21st Century*. Robert Wood Johnson Foundation. Princeton, NJ. https://publichealth.gwu.edu/sites/default/files/downloads/HPM/Activating%20Nursing%20To%20Address%20Unmet%20Needs%20In%20The%2021st%20Century.pdf.

Planetary Health Alliance. (n.d.). *Planetary health*. https://www.planetary-healthalliance.org/planetary-health.

Powers, M., & Faden, R. (2006). *Social justice: The moral foundations of public health and health policy*. New York, NY: Oxford University Press.

————. (2019). *Structural injustice: Power, advantage, and human rights*. New York, NY: Oxford University Press.

Public Health Accreditation Board (PHAB). (2014). Public Health Accreditation Board standards and measures. http://www.phaboard.org/about-phab/.

Public Health Foundation (PHF). (2014). *Core competencies for public health professionals*. Council on Linkages between academia and public health practice. phf.org/core competencies.

————. (2019). *Competencies for population health professionals*. http://www.phf.org/resourcestools/Documents/Population_Health_Competencies_2019Mar.pdf.

Public Health Leadership Society (PHLS). (2002). *Principles of ethical practice of public health, version 2.2*. https://www.apha.org/~/media/files/pdf/membergroups/ethics_brochure.ashx.

Public Health Nursing Section. (2001). *Public health interventions—Applications for public health nursing practice*. St. Paul: Minnesota Department of Health. https://www.health.state.mn.us/communities/practice/research/phncouncil/docs/0301wheel_manual.pdf.

Quad Council Coalition (QCC) Competency Review Task Force. (2018). Community/public health nursing competencies. https://www.cphno.org/wp-content/uploads/2020/08/QCC-C-PHN-COMPETENCIES-Approved_2018.05.04_Final-002.pdf.

Quad Council of Public Health Nursing Organizations. (1997). *The tenets of public health nursing*. Unpublished white paper.

Radzyminski, S. (2007). The concept of population health within the nursing profession. *Journal of Professional Nursing, 23*(1), 37–46.

Rawls, J. (1971). *A theory of justice*. Cambridge, MA: Harvard University Press.

Rentmeester, C. A., & Dasgupta, R. (2012). Good epidemiology, good ethics: Empirical and ethical dimensions of global public health. *Indian Journal of Medical Ethics, IX*(4), 235–241.

Robert Wood Johnson Foundation (RWJF). (2019). *Culture of health measures compendium measures update 2019*. https://www.rwjf.org/content/rwjf/en/culture-ofhealth/about/how-we-got-here.html#ten-underlying-principles.

————. (2021). *Building Culture of Health*. https://www.rwjf.org/en/how-we-work/building-a-culture-of-health.html#:~:text=The%20Robert%20Wood%20 Johnson%20Foundation,of%20our%20families%20and%20communities.

Shaw, K., Harpin, S., Steinke, G., Stember, M., & Krajicek, M. (2016). The DNP/ MPH dual degree: An innovative graduate education program for advanced public health nursing. *Public Health Nursing, 34*(2), 185–193.

Sherwin, S. (2008). Whither bioethics? How feminism can help reorient bioethics. *International Journal of Feminist Approaches to Bioethics, 1*(1), 7–27.

Siegel, A. W., & Merritt, M. M. (2019). An overview of conceptual foundations, ethical tensions, and ethical frameworks in public health. In A. C. Mastroianni, J. P. Kahn, & N. E. Kass (eds.), *The Oxford handbook of public health ethics* (5-11). New York, NY: Oxford University Press.

Siwicki, B. (2017). Advanced tech is evolving nursing education to meet hospital demand. *Health Care IT news*. https://www.healthcareitnews.com/news/advanced-tech-evolving-nursing-education-meet-hospital-demand.

Smith, C. (2013). Origins and future of community/public health nursing. In F. Maurer & C. Smith (eds.), *Community/Public health nursing practice: Health for families and populations* (31–53). St. Louis: Elsevier.

Srinivasan, S., & Williams, S. D. (2014). Transitioning from health disparities to a health equity research agenda: The time is now. *Public Health Reports, 129*(Supplement 2), 71–76.

Storfjell, J., Winslow, E., & Saunders, J. (2017). *Catalysts for change: Harnessing the power of nurses to build population health in the 21st century*. Princeton, NJ: Robert Wood Johnson Foundation. https://campaignforaction.org/resource/catalysts-change-harnessing-power-nurses-build-population-health-21st-century/.

Stringer, H. (2019). IOM future of nursing report card: Progress after 10 years. https://www.nurse.com/blog/2019/07/01/iom-future-of-nursing-report-card -progress-after-10-years/.

Summers, J. (2014). Theory of healthcare ethics. In E. E. Morrison & B. Furlong (eds.), *Health Care Ethics* (3–45). Burlington, MA: Jones and Bartlett.

Sun, A. (2019). Social justice leadership in urban schools: What do Black and Hispanic principals do to promote social justice? *Alberta Journal of Educational Research, 65*(2), 146–161.

Swider, S., Levin, P., & Reising, V. (2017). Evidence of public health nursing effectiveness: A realist review. *Public Health Nursing, 24*, 324–334. doi:10.1111/phn.12320.

Thrift, E., & Sugarman, J. (2019). What is social justice? Implications for psychology. *Journal of Theoretical and Philosophical Psychology, 39*(1), 1–17.

Toney-Butler, T., & Thayer, J. (2020). *Nursing process.* StatPearls Publishing. https://www.ncbi.nlm.nih.gov/books/NBK499937/.

University of Michigan Center for Excellence in Public Health Workforce Studies. (2013). *Enumeration and characterization of the public health nurse workforce: Findings of the 2012 public health nurse workforce surveys.* Ann Arbor, MI: University of Michigan. https://www.rwjf.org/content/dam/farm/reports/reports/2013/rwjf406659.

US Census Bureau. (2015). Projections of the size and composition of the U.S. population: 2014–2060. https://www.census.gov/library/publications/2015/demo/p25-1143.html.

US Environmental Protection Agency (USEPA). (2016). Management alert: Drinking water contamination in Flint, Michigan, demonstrates a need to clarify EPA authority to issue emergency orders to protect the public. Washington, DC: Office of Inspector General. No. 17-P-0004.

US Department of Health and Human Services. (1985). *Consensus conference on the essentials of public health nursing practice and education: Report of the conference.* Rockville, MD: Author.

Wabnitz, K-J., Gabrysch, S., Giunto, R., Haines, A., Herrmann, M., Howard, C., Potter, T., Prescott, S. L., & Redvers, N. (2020). A pledge for planetary health to unite health professionals in the Anthropocene. *Lancet, 396*(10261), 1471–1473.

Wallwork, E. (2008). Ethical analysis of research partnerships with communities. *Kennedy Institute of Ethics Journal, 18*(1), 57–85.

Watts, M. H., Michel, K. H., Breslin, J., & Tobin-Tyler, E. (2021). Equitable enforcement of pandemic-related public health laws: Strategies for achieving racial and health justice. *American Journal of Public Health, 111*(3), 395–397.

Whitmee, S., Haines, A., Beyrer, C., Boltz, F., Capon, A. G., de Souza Dias, B. F., Ezeb, A., Frumkin, H., Gong, P., Head, P., Horton, R., Mace, G. M., Marten, R., Myers, S. S., Nishtar, S., Ososfsky, S. A., Pattanayak, S. K., Pongsiri, M. J., Romanelli, C., Soucat, A., Vega, J., & Yach, D. (2015). Safeguarding human health in the Anthropocene epoch: Report of the Rockefeller Foundation–Lancet Commission on planetary health. *Lancet, 386*(10007), 1973–2028. doi:10.1016/S0140-6736(15)60901-1.

World Health Organization (WHO). (n.d.) *Social determinants of health.* https://www.who.int/health-topics/social-determinants-of-health#tab=tab_3

———. (2019a). About social determinants of health. https://www.who.int/social_determinants/en/.

———. (2019b). Health equity. Retrieved October 20, 2019, from https://www.who.int/topics/health_equity/en/.

———. (2021). Immunization coverage. https://www.who.int/news-room/factsheets/detail/immunization-coverage.

———. (2022). Health equity. https://www.who.int/health-topics/health-equity#tab=tab_1.

World Health Organization Eastern Mediterranean Regional Office (WHO EMRO). (2019). WHO EMRO: Health promotion and disease prevention through population-based interventions, including action to address social determinants and health inequity. http://www.emro.who.int/about-who/public-health-functions/health-promotion-disease-prevention.html.

Young, I. M. (1990). *Justice and the politics of difference.* Princeton, NJ: Princeton University Press.

———. (2011). *Responsibility for justice.* New York, NY: Oxford University Press.

Zotti, M., Brown, P., & Stotts, R. (1996). Community-based nursing versus community health nursing: What does it all mean? *Outlook, 44*(5), 211–217.

# Appendix A. Public Health Nursing: Past, Present, and Future

Public health nursing has evolved from the early days of Lillian Wald to present-day practice. Over time terms describing this practice have alternated between public health nursing to community health to accurately describe the focus on health across levels, but always within the context of the community.

The first known use of the term "public health nursing" is Lillian Wald's 1912 description of Public Health Nursing as the name for nurses "doing work for social betterment" in any setting (Brainard, 195; Fitzpatrick, 1975). The term "public" related to "all the people as a whole." By the 1920s the majority of public health nurses were employed by local and state health departments and the term "public" became associated with "employment by the government."

In the 1960s, the term *community health nursing* emerged to include nursing sponsored by private nonprofit organizations as well as government organizations (Hanlon & Pickett, 1984). Simultaneously, the American Nurses Association (ANA) created the Division of Community Health Nursing, which included nurses working in community-based settings (US Department of Health and Human Services [USDHHS], 1985). Therefore, the term *community health nursing* came to be associated with the *setting of practice* rather than the *focus of practice*. ANA published standards for nursing specialties in 1973, including *Standards of Community Health Nursing Practice*.

In 1986, ANA's Council of Community Health Nurses revised *Standards of Community Health Nursing Practice*. This publication explicitly states that "the terms *community health nurse* and *public health nurse* are synonymous" (American Nurses Association [ANA], 1986, p. 2). "Community health nursing practice promotes and preserves the health of populations by integrating the skills and knowledge relevant to both nursing and public health" (ANA, 1986, p. 1). Generalist community health nurses with baccalaureate degrees were to apply the nursing process with individuals, families, and groups. Specialist community health nurses with graduate degrees were to apply the nursing process with communities. Home health, occupational health, and school health were viewed as subspecialty areas of community health nursing.

By the 1990s, attempts were being made to distinguish community health nurses who had baccalaureate or higher education and experience in nursing and public health from other nurses who provided nursing in community settings, such as home health nurses (Baldwin et al., 1998; Smith, 2013; Zotti et al., 1996). Some organizations and authors used the term *community/public health nurse* to distinguish those community-based nurses who provide population-focused or community-focused care (Baldwin et al., 1998). Baldwin et al. (1998) recommended that the terms *community health* and *public health nursing* be abandoned, and "population-focused nursing or population health nursing" be used. Thus, the term *public* would be replaced by *population*. The Public Health Nursing Section of the Minnesota Department of Health retained the term *public health nursing* and asserted that the practice is "population-based public health practice" aimed at improving "the health status of entire identified populations" (2001, p. 7). The term *based* does not refer to physical setting but means "on which the care is founded" (Smith, 2013, p. 45).

In 1999, the Quad Council (QC) of Public Health Nursing Organizations and ANA published *Scope and Standards of Public Health Nursing Practice*. In that publication, PH nursing was described as "population-focused and community-oriented nursing practice" (ANA, 1999, p. 2). PH nursing was distinguished from community health nursing. Community-based care, which designates *site of care*, was stated to be a part of community-oriented care, which designates *focus of care*. PHNs were to ensure community-based care as a PN nursing strategy. "Public health nurses… [ensure] the availability of care to individuals and families in the community (community-based care) when their health condition creates a risk to the health of the population. Community-based care is a public health nursing strategy that directly benefits the whole population by reducing exposure to risk factors" (ANA, 1999, p. 5). The subsequent

2007 *Public Health Nursing: Scope and Standards of Practice* revision incorporated and replaced the 1986 *Standards of Community Health Nursing Practice.*

Since the turn of the 21st century, *public health nursing* has been the term used in ANA's *Public Health Nursing: Scope and Standards of Practice* (2007, 2013). The PH nursing scope and standards document recommends that all steps of the PH nursing process be applied with the population/community. Additionally, implementation can occur at multiple levels: individuals, families, groups, communities, and systems (ANA, 2013). Thus, PH nursing offers the expertise and leadership to promote the goals of *The Future of Nursing 2020–2030* and to advance the Culture of Health.

# Appendix B. PHN Workforce Data by Program Area and Job Function

**Table B.1. Program Areas of Registered Nurses in State and Local Health Departments (in order of survey designation).**

| State Health Department (SHD) | Local Health Department (LHD) |
| --- | --- |
| Inspections | Case management/care coordination |
| Family-planning services | Communicable disease |
| Home health care | School health |
| Communicable disease | Immunizations |
| Case management/care coordination | Family-planning services |
| Maternal and child health programs | Home health care |
| General administration | Administration |
| Access to care | Ambulatory service |
| Chronic disease services | WIC |
| Women, Infant, Children Supplemental Nutrition Program (WIC) | Chronic disease services |
| Emergency preparedness | Emergency preparedness |
| School health | Access to care |
| Substance abuse services | Inspections |
| Ambulatory services | Correctional health |
| Refugee health | Substance abuse services |
| Correctional health | Environmental health |
| Other | Other |
| Infection Control | |

**Table B.2. Job Functions of Registered Nurses in State and Local Health Departments (in order of survey designation).**

| SHD | LHD |
|---|---|
| Clinic-based care | Clinic-based care |
| Administration/staff supervision | Community engagement |
| Outreach activities | Administration/staff supervision |
| Population-level prevention | Outreach activities |
| Quality improvement initiatives | Population-level prevention |
| Community engagement | Quality improvement initiatives |
| Workforce development activities | Workforce development activities |

©2013 University of Michigan. *Enumeration and Characterization of the Public Health Nurse Workforce: Findings of the 2012 Public Health Nurse Workforce Surveys Center of Excellence in Public Health Workforce Studies*, Ann Arbor, MI.

# Appendix C. Certifications Relevant to Public Health Nursing Practice

| Exam | Credentialing Body | Eligibility |
|------|-------------------|-------------|
| Certified Public Health Exam (CPH) Implemented 2008 | National Board of Public Health Examiners | Bachelors or above and five or more years of work experience Student/graduate of Council on Education for Public Health– (CEPH-) accredited school/program |
| Certification in Infection Control (CIC) | Certification Board of Infection Control and Epidemiology (CBIC) | Completed postsecondary education in a health-related field, including but not limited to medicine, nursing, laboratory technology, or public health Recommended two years of experience in infection prevention and control, which includes experience in these specific areas |
| Certified Health Education Specialist (CHES) Implemented 1989 | National Commission for Health Education Credentialing, Inc | Bachelors or above in health education or related degree and 25 credits in health education |

**(Continued)**

| Exam | Credentialing Body | Eligibility |
|---|---|---|
| Certified Correctional Health Professional – Registered Nurse (CCHP-RN) | National Commission on Correctional Health Care | Prerequisite – registered nurses (RN) must first apply, pass exam, and be certified in CCHP. To apply for the CCHP-RN, the RN must have practiced the equivalent of two years full-time as a registered nurse, have a minimum of 2,000 hours in a correctional setting in the last three years, and have completed 54 hours of continuing education, including at least 18 hours in correctional nursing within the last three years. CCHP-RN certification requires the completion of an application and a passing score on a two-hour, proctored, multiple-choice examination. https://www.ncchc.org/CCHP-RN |
| Master Certified Health Education Specialist (MCHES) Implemented 2011 | National Commission for Health Education Credentialing, Inc. | Five or more years as CHES or master's and above with five or more years of experience |
| Informatics Nursing Certification (RN-BC) | American Nurses Credentialing Center | Hold a current, active RN license in a state or territory of the US or hold the professional, legally recognized equivalent in another country |
| | | Hold a bachelor's or higher degree in nursing or a bachelor's degree in a relevant field |
| | | Have practiced the equivalent of two years full-time as a registered nurse |
| | | Have completed 30 hours of continuing education in informatics nursing within the last three years |
| | | Meet practice hour requirements |

*(Continued)*

| Exam | Credentialing Body | Eligibility |
|---|---|---|
| Nurse Executive Certification (NE-BC) | American Nurses Credentialing Center | Hold a current, active RN license in a state or territory of the US or hold the professional, legally recognized equivalent in another country<br><br>Hold a bachelor's or higher degree in nursing<br><br>Have held a mid-level administrative or higher position (e.g., nurse manager, supervisor, director, assistant director) OR a faculty position teaching graduate students/nursing administration OR a nursing management or executive consultation position full-time for at least 24 months (or the equivalent) in the last five years<br><br>Have completed 30 hours of continuing education in nursing administration within the last three years (this requirement is waived if you have a master's degree in nursing administration) |
| Nurse Executive Advanced Certification (NEA-BC) | American Nurses Credentialing Center | Hold a current, active RN license in a state or territory of the US or hold the professional, legally recognized equivalent in another country<br><br>Hold a master's or higher degree in nursing or hold a bachelor's degree in nursing and a master's in another field<br><br>Have held an administrative position at the nurse executive level or a faculty position teaching graduate students executive-level nursing administration full-time for at least 24 months (or the equivalent) in the last five years<br><br>Have completed 30 hours of continuing education in nursing administration within the last three years (this requirement is waived if you hold a master's degree in nursing administration) |

**(Continued)**

| Exam | Credentialing Body | Eligibility |
| --- | --- | --- |
| Nursing Case Management Certification | American Nurses Credentialing Center | Hold a current, active RN license or equivalent in another country |
| | | Two years of experience as RN |
| | | Completion of 2,000 hours of case management experience in last three years |
| | | Completion of 30 hours of continuing education in nursing case management in three years |
| Nationally Certified School Nurse (NCSN) | National Board for Certification of School Nurses | A bachelor's degree or higher **in nursing** or the equivalent in other countries |
| | | A bachelor's degree or higher in a **health-related field relevant to school nursing** |
| | | Candidates with a bachelor's degree or higher in a **non-nursing or non-health-related field** must have a total of six additional credits for undergraduate or graduate courses in any combination of the following subjects: |
| | | 1. Management of primary health care problems of children and/ or adolescents |
| | | 2. Health assessment of children and/ or adolescents |
| | | 3. Public health/community health/ epidemiology |
| | | OR |
| | | Current certification by NBCSN as an NCSN |
| | | 1,000 hours clinical practice requirements within three years |

# Index

Clinical interventions, 28

Clinic's fliers, 44

*Code of Ethics for Nurses with Interpretive Statements 2015,* 39

Codes of ethics, 39

Collaboration, 1, 2, 6, 8, 11, 20, 22, 24, 25, 27, 30, 31, 36, 54, 57, 61, 64, 69, 72, 78, 95–99, 108

Communicable diseases, 60

Communication, 11, 22, 23, 44, 51, 61, 69, 81, 91, 93, 94, 96

Community, 1–13, 7, 17, 19, 21, 23, 25, 27, 29, 31, 36, 40, 41, 48, 54, 58, 64, 67, 71, 73, 76, 78, 81, 82, 88, 89, 95, 100, 104, 105

Community-based care, 130

Community-based participatory research (CBPR), 31–32, 78

Community collaboration, 6. *See also* Collaboration

Community engagement (CE), 30, 71

*the Community Guide,* 67

Community health, 130

Community health assessment (CHA), 9, 55. *See also* Assessment

Community health nursing, 2, 3

Community health workers (CHW), 44

Community/public health nursing competencies, 23–24

Community-wide syndromic surveillance, 60

Competence evaluation, components of, 50

Competence, evaluation of, 49–51

Competencies, 70, 71. *See also* Standards of practice

Competency evaluation instruments, 52–53

Consultation, 82

Coordination of care, 79

Coordination of disaster health services and shelters, 60

Core functions of public health, 18–19

COVID-19, 41, 43, 60, 61, 63

COVID-19 vaccine, 43

CPH. *See* Certified Public Health Exam (CPH)

Credentialing body, 134–137

Credibility, 51

Cultural competence, 11

Cultural heritage, 11

Cultural humility, 11, 12

Culturally congruent practice, 11–12

Cultural safety, 12

Cultural sensitivity, 11

Culture of health, 24

## D

Data collection, 72, 73, 80

Deaths, 60

Decision-making processes, 6

Deontology, 13

Diagnoses, 35, 73

Disabilities, 7

Disaster recovery, 26–27

Disparities, 5, 17, 45, 62, 63, 65, 67, 71, 89

DNP programs, 59

Dock, Lavinia, 1

Doctor of Nursing Practice (DNP), 58

Documentation, 74

Drug-resistant organisms, 60

Drug-resistant tuberculosis, 61

Dynamic nature of public health nursing, 17

## E

Ebola virus, 61

Ecological model of health, 10–11

Ecological perspective, 71, 73, 79, 105, 107

Education, 3–5, 11, 13, 14, 16–18, 22, 25, 27, 28, 30, 32, 33, 37, 42, 46, 47, 49, 53, 55–59, 61, 64–70, 69, 81, 82, 99

Educational standards, 58

Education for public health nursing roles, 64

Electronic health record (EHR), 48

Eligibility, 134–137

Emergency management services (EMS), 27